Educational Audiology
for the
Hard of Hearing Child

Educational Audiology for the Hard of Hearing Child

Frederick S. Berg, Ph.D.
Professor

James C. Blair, Ph.D.
Associate Professor

Steven H. Viehweg, Ph.D.
Associate Professor

Ann Wilson-Vlotman, Ed.D.
Coordinator of Project Intervention

Department of Communicative Disorders
Utah State University, Logan Utah

Grune & Stratton, Inc.
Harcourt Brace Jovanovich, Publishers
Orlando   New York   San Diego   Boston   London
San Francisco   Tokyo   Sydney   Toronto

Grune & Stratton, Inc.
Orlando, Florida 32887

Distributed in the United Kingdom by
Grune & Stratton, Ltd.
24/28 Oval Road, London NW 1

Library of Congress Catalog Number 85-081927
International Standard Book Number 0-8089-1771-4
Printed in the United States of America
85 86 87 88 89   10 9 8 7 6 5 4 3 2 1

492608

Contents

Preface

This book describes the state-of-art in educational audiology, a main branch of both the audiological and educational professions. The book deals with hearing impaired children, particularly youngsters enrolled in the regular public schools and especially hard of hearing children.

With the passage of the All Handicapped Children's Act in 1975, a need for the specialty of educational audiology became professionally recognized. Since then professional training programs in audiology, education of the hearing impaired, and speech-language pathology have provided increasing coursework and practicum focused on the characteristics and needs of hearing impaired children in the regular schools. The literature of educational audiology has been growing accordingly.

The current book is the third of a series of books on educational audiology written at Utah State University. The first book, *The Hard of Hearing Child,* was printed in 1970. The second book, *Educational Audiology,* was printed in 1976. The present book describes earlier as well as recent developments and sets the stage for a new round of improvements in the state-of-the art.

This book includes eight interrelated chapters. The characteristics of hard of hearing children and the service needs of hearing impaired children in the regular schools are covered in Chapters 1 and 2. A model for the delivery of services by the educational audiologist, based on a recent national survey, is introduced. A new assessment model is covered at length in Chapter 3. In Chapters 4 and 5 audiological considerations and hearing aids for school children are described. Chapters 6 and 7 detail listening and speech programs as well as classroom acoustics and signal amplification and transmission equipment. The final chapter (8) describes the changing roles of parents, teachers, and school administrators in meeting the needs of hard of hearing children in regular classrooms, and the responsibilities of educational audiologists in the change process.

Four educational audiologists have collaborated in the planning and writing of this book. The uniqueness of separate personalities as well as common purpose is hopefully evident. Each contributor is a member of the recently organized Educational Audiology Association.

Frederick S. Berg

1
Characteristics of the Target Population

This chapter addresses the characteristics and deficiencies of hard-of-hearing students in the elementary and secondary schools of our nation. Initially, the prevalence of this target population and the unsolved problem of identifying students with hearing loss are described. Next, the various underlying ear pathologies are briefly reviewed. The remainder of the chapter covers deficiencies of hard-of-hearing students, beginning with listening problems and ending with vocational problems. The following chapters also focus on hard-of-hearing students, but consider as well the deaf who are mainstreamed.

TARGET POPULATION

Hearing loss is one of the most prevalent handicapping conditions. By the age of two, 75 percent of children have had at least one espisode of otitis media, which is only one of many etiologies which can cause hearing loss (Richardson & Donaldson, 1981). Between kindergarten and 12th grade, approximately one in every five children has a conductive, sensory, neural, or mixed hearing loss in one or both ears, stemming from one of many etiologies.* Table 1-1 presents hearing threshold data on a 38,568-person national sample of males and females; this data was obtained in mobile testing units by audiologists employed by Colorado State University.

Currently only a minority of the entire school population is systematically tested for hearing loss. Equipment, facilities, and techniques could be made

---

*Personal Communication from J Willeford, Colorado State Universtiy, Fort Collins, Colorado, January 25, 1971.

Table 1-1.
Number of school-age children with varying unilateral and
bilateral hearing impairment for each 1000 youngsters from a
38,568-child sample of all youngsters in the elementary and
secondary schools of the United States

dB Loss	Unilateral	Bilateral
11–25 (slight)	154 +	34
26–45 (mild)	13 +	5
46–100 + (moderate-severe-profound)	3 +	2

available for accomplishing a mass program for evaluation of hearing losses
in the schools, but educational resources have not been marshalled for such
a task. Consequently, only the children with the most obvious hearing losses
tend to be earmarked for special support. Data from Table 1-1 indicates that
more than 8 million of the 39.5 million children in the schools have hearing
loss, but national summaries of handicapped children receiving special education and related services reveals that only about 41,000 hard-of-hearing
children and 41,000 deaf children have been singled out for extra consideration. Only about one child in every 100 hearing impaired children in the
regular and special schools of the country is therefore receiving special
educational support (Feistritzer, 1983, p. 7; United States Department of
Education, 1980†).

The most frequently occurring hearing problem among school children
is conductive loss from active ear disease, but this problem is not being
uncovered on a widespread basis. Every other child with a conductive hearing
loss is missed when tested by the traditional 25-decibel (25-dB) pure-tone
screening often exclusively used. A newer technique, recommended for use
together with pure-tone screening, is impedence screening, but it has yet to
reach the schools in a major way. Consequently, the great majority of children
with hearing loss, particularly those with the least unilateral and bilateral
involvement, are often left unidentified. Without comprehensive hearing
screening and testing, the task of identification is very difficult.

The hearing impaired child has the same physical appearance as his friends
who have normal hearing; he also behaves essentially as they do. Even his
disabilities may be easily misunderstood as merely negative variations of normal
behavior. For example, when the teacher of a child with a hearing defect speaks
to him one time, he may be watching her and—with what he receives from
hearing reinforced by what he receives from sight—responds correctly. Another
time when she speaks, the background noise may cover too much of what she
says for him to decode the message correctly, or he may miss some of the

†Personal Communication from J. Rosenstein. Report of handicapped children receiving
special education and related services as reported by state agenices under P.L. 94–142 and P.L.
89–313, school year 1979–80. July 21, 1980.

essential cues from her face if it is turned away from him. This time he misunderstands and responds erroneously. His behavior is thus erratic depending upon such factors as the auditory characteristics of his hearing and of the background noises, manner with which the teacher speaks, and her position relative to his view, in addition to the random variations found in any child. But then, the child with normal hearing is often inattentive or distracted by other events and, therefore, is erratic in his responses to spoken language. For this reason the teacher is likely to interpret the intermittency in performance of the hard-of-hearing child to lack of self-descipline. When he does "pay attention," he seems to "get along fine." (Fletcher, 1970, p.4.)

Parents and teachers may know that the child has had an ear infection or another etiology that can lead to hearing loss, but may not really know if a temporary or permanent hearing loss exists unless regular audiometric testing is performed. When a child has a severe or profound hearing loss, a parent typically makes the diagnosis of hearing loss before the child is 2 years old, although the family doctor or pediatrician might tend to negate this finding (Fellendorf, 1975, p. 11). The child with a less severe hearing loss poses a more difficult identification problem, particularly during the early years of life and school. This child responds to sound, but inconsistently, and develops speech and language, but slowly and imperfectly. When parents and teachers are not oriented to the differences between deaf and hard-of-hearing children, they behave as does the general public and tend to think of deafness as an all-or-nothing phenomenon (Boothroyd, 1982, p. 66).

The problem of identifying hard-of-hearing children extends from the preschool years through the elementary and secondary school years. The specific task is to distinguish the hard-of-hearing child from the normally hearing child and from the deaf child. One purpose of this recognition is simply to take a first step in providing appropriate educational services for the hard of hearing. In the past, the hard-of-hearing child has tended to be educated as either a normal hearing youngster or as a deaf child, without due consideration being given to the varying communication abilities of these 3 populations. Communicatively, the hard-of-hearing child is more like the normal hearing child than like the deaf child, because both use audition rather than vision as the primary mode for speech and language development and usage. However, the hard-of-hearing child will be neglected in both the regular class and the special class for the deaf unless recognition is given to that child's unique communication problems.

The measurement of hearing contributes to the differentiation of the hard-of-hearing child from the normal hearing child and from the deaf child. If the child has a hearing loss for speech in the better ear of 15 dB or less, that child often can be considered a normal hearing child. If the hearing loss is 16 dB or greater, the child can be called hard of hearing, unless the loss is so great that audition is no longer the primary communicative input mode. On the average, 95–100 dB is a dividing line between being hard of hearing and being deaf (Ross, 1982, pp. 3–4). When hearing loss is great, however, determining whether a specific child is hard of hearing or deaf depends on more than reference to the 95–100 dB cutoff. In schools or classes for the deaf, for example, about half of the children have less than a 95-dB hearing loss, and yet these children tend to function as deaf children because their residual hearing has not been fully utilized (Ross 1982, p. 3; Wedenberg, 1981). If we do not identify which children can function as hard of hearing rather than deaf, we are ignoring a potential for speech and language development and functioning that can expand the communicative world for many hearing-impaired children. This is not to put down the deaf child who must rely primarily upon vision (lipreading, visual cues, or manual communication) for communication, and who often can use audition as a significant secondary or supplementary communicative mode. Currently, however, we are not tapping the residual hearing capabilities of either the deaf or hard of hearing to the extent that is possible and even practical. Educators should not neglect either of these subpopulations of hearing-impaired children.

EAR PATHOLOGY

Hearing loss is organic or functional. An organic hearing loss has a physical basis, whereas a functional hearing loss is psychological in origin. Organic hearing loss constitutes nearly all hearing loss among children (Newby, 1979, p. 62). A specific pathology or lesion of organic hearing loss affects one or more of the 3 components of the hearing mechanism: conductive, sensory, or neural. The conductive component includes the outer and middle ears, the sensory component the 2 cochleas, and the neural component the auditory nerves and all those parts of the brain concerned with the processing of auditory information. The outer and middle ears conduct sound from the surrounding air to the cochleas and protect them from the effects of loud noises and direct physical damage. Each cochlea, called an end organ of hearing, converts the physical characterisitcs of sound into corresponding neural information which the brain can process and interpret. Each side of the brain receives information from both the right and left ears. (Boothroyd, 1982, pp. 13–16).

Hearing pathology or disorder results from various genetic defects, diseases, drugs, or traumas. These general causes and specific examples have been summarized (Boothroyd, 1982, p.50). The type of loss (conductive, sensory, or neural), time acquired, degree of loss, stability, and occurrence of additional impairments are specified. Almost twice as many specific etiologies result in sensory (cochlear) hearing loss than in either conductive or neural hearing loss. The most common causes of conductive hearing loss, namely impacted wax in the outer ear and otitis media, result in lesser degrees of hearing loss which fluctuate over time. Most other etiologies, including genetic factors and rubella, result in mild-to-profound hearing impairment. Most hearing loss is acquired rather than congenital. About half of the etiologies resulting in hearing loss can lead to additional impairments, including perceptual or symbolic dysfunction. The population of hearing-impaired children, both hard of hearing and deaf, presents a wide variety of characteristics and needs.

DEFICIENCIES OF THE HARD OF HEARING

The hard-of-hearing child presents a bewildering complexity of problems to consider. These problems encompass listening, speech, language, cognition and academics, emotions and social relations, parental and societal reactions, and vocational performance.

Listening Problem

Broadly defined, listening is the decoding of any auditory stimulus, whether it be an environmental sound or a person speaking. The definition needs to be broadened to encompass the perception of speech through audition, vision (speech-reading or lipreading), or both in combination. We have all had the experience of having to look at a person in order to understand what was being said when the person was speaking from a distance or in the presence of noise (Berg, 1978, p. 1).

Listening efficiency depends upon many variables of the speaker, listener, environment, and speech code. Whereas the normal hearing child can usually perceive the entirety of speech if it is not too faint or too far away, the hard-of-hearing child typically decodes less of the spoken message. If the child has a conductive impairment, speech will be faint or may not be heard.

A simple test for experiencing the listening impact of just a slight conductive bilateral hearing loss has been described by Downs (1981):

> With your fingers extended, press the tabs in front of your ears into the ear canals, occluding the ear canals completely. Press tightly. You have just given yourself a 25 dB HL average hearing loss... Try carrying on a normal conversation with this hearing loss, or try listening to someone talk in a crowd. You will find that you have to strain a great deal in order to catch what people are saying. (Downs, 1981, p. 177).

When sensory (cochlear) impairment exists, speech might not only be difficult to detect but to discriminate, even if made loud enough. Likewise, if the neural mechanism is damaged close to the cochlea, loss of sensitivity and discrimination might be evident. With a mild discrimination problem, similar words such as *track* and *trap* sound alike. When a discrimination problem is severe, words as dissimilar as *pig* and *doll* may not be differentiated, nor might two very different environmental sounds. If the lesion is in the brain stem or at a still higher level, the child may have difficulties also with auditory attention, awareness, memory, or association (Boothroyd, 1982).

Speech reception can break down at various listening levels: detection, discrimination, identification or recognition, and comprehension.

> Detection is the ability to perceive the presence of an acoustic event; discrimination, to hear the difference between one sound and another; identification, to recognize one sound pattern as distinct from all others; and comprehension, to understand the meaning of the speech signal (Ling, 1981).

Listening levels or subprocesses are clarified if related to questions such as: "Was there a sound?" (detection); "Was this sound different from that sound?" (discrimination); "What was the sound like?" (sensation); "Where did the sound originate?" (localization); "What made the sound?" (recognition); and "Why was the sound made?" (comprehension) (Boothroyd, 1982, pp. 17–20).

Hard-of-hearing children often do not comprehend speech because they do not have the potential for detecting, discriminating, sensing, localizing, or recognizing as much information as do normal hearing children. Hard-of-hearing children are more dependent upon a redundancy of information being provided by the speaker, the speech signal, or the environment to counteract breakdown in speech reception. For example, room noise may need to be reduced or lipreading may need to be added to residual hearing in order for the hard-of-hearing child to comprehend speech (Sanders, D., 1982, pp. 27–30).

Normally there is a comfortable redundancy of clues for decoding speech messages.

> When we listen under favorable conditions, the clues available are far in excess of what is actually needed for satisfactory recognition. Indeed, general context is often so compelling that we know positively what is going to be said even before we hear the words. This is why under normal conditions we understand speech with ease and certainty, despite the ambiguities of acoustic cues. It is also the reason that intelligibility is maintained to such an astonishing extent, despite the variability of speakers, in the presence of noise and distortion (Denes & Pinson, 1963, p. 146).

Many professionals have previously held the widespread view that children with unilateral hearing loss have problems localizing where sound is coming from, but that, with preferential seating, they compensate for speech recognition problems. A recent study by Bess (1982) challenges this basic assumption. Bess compared both the localization and syllable recognition performance of 25 children with moderate-to-profound unilateral hearing loss to that of a matched group of normal hearing listeners. The children with unilateral hearing loss not only made more localization errors than did their normal hearing counterparts, but they also scored lower in syllable recognition tasks. The lower recognition scores occurred under conditions simulating regular seating and preferential seating. In the first condition, noise was presented to the good ear and speech to the impaired ear. In the second condition, which simulated preferential seating, the syllables were presented to the good ear and noise to the poor ear. Bess concluded that-(1) the greater the hearing loss the poorer the localization ability; and, (2) the more adverse the listening condition the poorer the speech recognition.

Children with either unilateral or bilateral hearing loss may have problems listening in typical school classrooms. Competing noise and, at times, excessive reverberation interfere with speech reception by masking and smearing speech, respectively. The classroom acoustics problem will be discussed further in Chapter 7.

While a unilateral hearing loss presents a definite listening problem to the child, a bilateral hearing impairment results in a more extensive listening breakdown. A bilateral loss causes part of the sound environment to be shut out of both cochleas and both auditory nerves. Bilateral hearing loss has such an evident impact upon listening that classifications of hearing handicap in the literature are based almost entirely upon the assumption that a lesion exists in both ears (Davis, H., 1978). A hearing handicap classification should reflect, however, various degrees of both unilateral and bilateral hearing losses. An example of such a classification based on speech detection appears below.

If children cannot detect sound, they cannot localize, recognize, or comprehend it. Detection is the lowest level of the auditory reception hierarchy. Detection loss is expressed in decibels and occurs when a lesion is in any site of the auditory mechanism, or when hearing loss is conductive, sensory, neural, or central in origin. The effects of just a detection or decibel loss are below hypothetically related to categories of unilateral and bilateral hearing loss. It is assumed that the child is listening in a typical classroom environment at 12 feet distant from the sound source and without a hearing aid.

- *Slight unilateral, 11–25 dB.* Faint sounds from impaired-ear side of head tend not to be detected.
- *Mild Unilateral, 26–45 dB.* Faint sounds from impaired-ear side of head are not detected.
- *Moderate to profound unilateral, 46–100+ dB.* Conversational level sounds from impaired-ear side of head tend not to be detected.
- *Slight bilateral, 11–25 dB.* Faint sounds from better-ear side of head tend not to be detected.
- *Mild bilateral, 26–45 dB.* Faint sounds from better-ear side of head are not detected.
- *Moderate to profound bilateral, 46–100+ dB.* Conversational level to loud level sounds from better-ear side of head tend not to be detected or are not detected.

The speech detection problem of unilateral and bilateral hearing loss is accompanied by corresponding loss of environmental awareness. Normally, the lead senses of audition and vision reach out to intercept acoustic and optical stimuli and keep a child in homeostasis with the close and distant environment as needed (Myklebust, 1960, pp. 46–48). Binaural hearing, a benefit of an intact auditory mechanism, is particularly adept at scanning the environment for meaningful events because of its multidirectional and depth-perception capabilities. With hearing loss, the child loses contact with certain sounds of the surrounding environment and loses the capacity to localize the origin of other sounds. Typically, with unilateral or bilateral hearing loss, the two ears of the child differ in speech detection sensitivity. Often, the less sensitive the child's hearing, the smaller the environmental field that can be detected or localized by the auditory mechanism. Pure-tone and speech detection thresholds for each ear are measured to provide data for estimating loss of environmental input in general and speech input in particular.

The pure-tone thresholds in decibels are plotted on an audiogram form for both ears of a child. Thresholds are often obtained for 7 octave intervals from 125 to 8000 Hertz (Hz), spanning the frequency range of the speech signal. The thresholds for the frequencies 500, 1000, and 2000 Hz may be averaged to arrive at a single decibel hearing loss for each ear. Based on this procedure, ranges of average thresholds have been arbitrarily determined, such as 0–15, 16–25, 26–40, 41–55, 56–70, 71–90, and 91–110 dB. The better-ear average threshold is used to affix corresponding terms expressing normal hearing or hearing loss of various degrees: *within normal, minimal* (slight), *mild, moderate, moderately severe, severe,* and *profound,* respectively (Rupp & Stockell, 1980).

The audiogram is the single most valuable audiometric data kept on a child; of all measures of hearing level that can be obtained, the audiogram seems to correlate most highly with the other measures. It is not, however, really closely correlated with any other single audiometric measure. Ling (1976, pp. 23–26) states that the audiogram merely indicates the dividing line between detecting the presence of sound and not detecting it, much as a shoreline divides land from water. A shoreline, however, does not describe the water behind it, just as an audiogram does not describe how well a child hears at suprathreshold intensities.

Often, we attempt to determine how well a hard-of-hearing child can perceive speech at a suprathreshold comfortable loudness level. The measurement of speech discrimination, recognition, or comprehension is, however, often clouded by the child's deficient speech and language and limited ability to write responses to speech stimuli. The speech perception data that we do have on hard-of-hearing children reveal that if they have nonconductive impairment, they do not discriminate, recognize, or comprehend speech as accurately as do normal hearing children, even when it is comfortably loud enough for them. In one study using the Word Intelligibility by Picture Identification (WIPI) test for children (Ross & Lerman, 1970), 21 children with moderate-to-severe hearing loss achieved a mean discrimination score of 59 percent. In another study using more conventional monosyllabic word lists, 12 children with mild-to-moderate loss achieved an average recognition score of 66 percent (Byers, 1973). The difficulty level of these 2 measures is, however, different because the WIPI test provides a measure of speech discrimination and the more conventional test provides a measure of speech recognition or identification. It is easier to point to a picture corresponding to a spoken word, from 6 options for each item on the WIPI test than to repeat each of 50 words of a monosyllabic list. Both test scores, however, measure generally depressed speech perception performance.

A breakdown of speech discrimination errors often made by children with moderate-to-profound bilateral hearing losses is presented below. Children with moderate or severe losses usually discriminate prosodic features, most vowels, voicing versus non-voicing, and manners of articulation. They confuse, however, consonants within articulatory groups or places of articulation. For example, when responding to words with initial /p/ within the Fairbanks Rhyme Speech Discrimination Test, Byers subjects substituted /t/ 16 percent, /k/ 15 percent, /f/ 7 percent, /s/ 8 percent, and /h/ 7 percent, for a total of 59 percent. In contrast, children with profound loss often have great difficulty in auditory discrimination of any of the prosodic or articulatory features of speech, with the exception of distinguishing nasal from non-nasal sounds and changes in speech intensity as a function of time (Erber, 1982, pp. 21–24).

A child with moderate-to-profound bilateral hearing impairment typically hears sound in a distorted way, particularly when not using an appropriate hearing aid. Often the child has an audiogram that indicates relatively less-sensitive hearing at the higher frequencies. In addition, intense speech input may be perceived as disproportionately loud. In the first instance, there is frequency distortion, and in the second instance, harmonic distortion. Both conditions interfere with speech discrimination and are evident with nonconductive hearing impairment.

Speech Problem

There is a lower incidence of speech problems than listening problems among the hard-of-hearing population. This is because most hard-of-hearing children have unilateral loss, or, if they have bilateral loss, they can still hear themselves well even if they cannot hear others as well. Speech development is somewhat delayed but not necessarily defective by the time the hard-of-hearing child has completed elementary school. The hard-of-hearing child has enough opportunities to hear others speak at close range to compensate for missed opportunities to listen at a distance. Distance, competing noise, and reverberation factors that continue to complicate the listening process do not have nearly as much impact upon speech development. Once speech behavior has been developed, it can be maintained through habit patterns that have been laid down in the brain, and it is minimally dependent upon sensory feedback (Ling, 1976, p. 4, pp. 66–73).

The presence or extent of a speech problem in a hard-of-hearing child is also influenced by whether hearing loss is congenital or adventitious, and by whether it is temporary or permanent, and by whether or not it is progressive. The more hearing the child has and the longer the child's hearing is at full capacity during the early years of life, the better the child's speech will be. With these considerations in mind, the absence or presence of a speech problem will be discussed for several categories of unilateral and bilateral hearing loss described earlier.

If a child has a unilateral hearing loss, ordinarily there is no speech problem manifest. The one good ear provides the needed signal input for speech modeling, development, and maintenance.

Most children with slight or mild bilateral hearing loss also learn to speak precisely or nearly so, although usually they are delayed in the acquisition of speech. When these children have conductive hearing loss, their final speech prognosis tends to be better than for those with other types of loss because they can discriminate and recognize sounds accurately when they can hear them. A child with sensory, neural, or central hearing loss may still ultimately exhibit blurred speech.

It is the children with moderate-to-profound bilateral deficit who account for most speech problems among the hard of hearing. These children have sensory, neural, or central hearing impairments that interfere substantially with the speech developmental processes during early childhood. In special education programs of the United States, intelligibility ratings have been used to judge the speech of hard-of-hearing children in this subcategory and comparison has been made to speech ratings of deaf children. In a 1974 study of 978 hearing-impaired children, for example, 90 percent of children with a hearing loss of 55 dB or less in the better ear were rated intelligible or very intelligible, whereas only 3 percent of children with hearing loss greater than 91 dB were rated very intelligible (Trybus, 1980).

DiCarlo (1968) studied the speech errors of 15 hard-of-hearing teenagers with a mean hearing loss of 60 dB and a mean speech recognition score of 34 percent. Remediation from early age had enabled these youngsters to develop normal sentence skills. Table 1-2 summarizes the percentages of 15 types of speech errors made by this hard-of-hearing sample. The three most common types of errors were misarticulation of consonant blends, misarticulation of arresting consonants, and nasalization of vowels.

West and Weber (1973) describe the phonology of a 4-year-old girl with a 58-dB loss in her better ear. The speech analysis was made from spontaneous language samples. Half of the utterances were intelligible. The /b/, /m/, /p/, /w/, /n/, /k/, and /h/ were correct more than 75 percent of the time;

Table 1-2.
Percentages of speech errors among hard-of-hearing teenagers

Type of Error	Percentage of Occurrence
1. Consonant omission	2.5
2. Regular consonant substitution	8.3
3. Breath-voice consonant substitiution	7.9
4. Consonant blend	20.8
5. Abutting consonant	3.1
6. Releasing consonant	3.0
7. Arresting consonant	24.1
8. Nasalization of consonant	1.6
9. Substitution of vowel	9.0
10. Dipthong fractionization	8.3
11. Diphthongization of vowel	2.2
12. Neutralization of vowel	0.4
13. Nasalization of vowel	34.4
14. Abnormal rhythm (prosody)	8.0
15. Arythmic sentence	1.3

the /d/. /tʃ/, /f/, /r/, /y/, /l/, and /t/ more than 50 percent but less than 75 percent of the time; and the /g/, /d/, /v/, /ð/, /z/, /ʃ/, /ʒ/, /ŋ/, /s/, and /θ/ were not present. Clearly, visible sounds occur often among the first group, tongue-tip sounds among the second group, and the normally most difficult articulations dominate the third group. This child showed a normal pattern of development in moving from easier to more difficult articulations, but speech acquisition was substantially retarded.

The order in which consonant sounds occurred in the phonology of the child with a moderate hearing loss just described may be compared with the order of normal consonant sound acquisition. Table 1-3 summarizes the order of normal consonant sound proficiency based on 50 percent of correct articulation for a sound in two out of three word positions (Sanders, E., 1972). By 4 years of age, the normal phonemic system is well on its way to being established (Eisenson & Ogilvie, 1983, pp. 161–162).

Children with moderate-to-profound bilateral hearing loss also tend to have some problem with vowel targets. The greater the hearing loss the

Table 1-3.
Normal order of consonant sound acquisition

Age in Years	Consonant sounds
2	h, m, n, w, b, p, t, k, g, n, d
3	f, y, j, s, r, l
4	tʃ, ʃ, dʒ, z, v
5	θ, ð
6	ʒ

greater the difficulty, as a rule. Depending on the severity of ear pathology, these children have more difficulty perceiving the frequency location of vowel formants and so more often perceptually confuse either (1) vowels produced in neighboring articulatory positions or (2) front and back vowels with similar first formants. Examples of these 2 problems are the confusion of /i/ and /ɪ/ or /i/ and /u/, respectively (Erber, 1980).

When a hard-of-hearing child has a speech problem, it characteristically involves articulation, sometimes involves nasality, and still less often involves refined control of intonation. Nasality reveals that velopharyngeal valving is defective, which can result from absence of the refined auditory feedback needed to regulate the fine nuances of nasality control. An intonation problem characteristically results from poor frequency discrimination. A 1–2 percent frequency discrimination is required to discriminate between two neighboring tones. Children with severe bilateral hearing losses in the 70–90 dB range vary in frequency discrimination from 2 to 30 percent, which is normal to moderately poor (Risberg, Agelfors, & Boberg, 1975).

In contrast to the child with the type of hearing loss just described, the deaf child has a greater articulation, nasality, and intonation problem, and, additionally, voice and timing and rhythm deficits, even after speech intervention (Nickerson, 1975). At the same time, a normally hearing child between five and seven years of age has precise timing and rhythm, pitch and intonation, velar control, articulation, and voice quality. The speech behavior of the hard-of-hearing child tends therefore to be more like that of the normal hearing child than that of the deaf child.

In summary, the speech of children with bilateral hearing loss who are not deaf is often characteristic of the speech of much younger normally hearing children (Ross, p. 17 1982). In contrast, "the speech of deaf children differs from normal speech in all regards" (Black, 1971). The speech of the hard of hearing nevertheless constitutes a formidable problem in that it may interfere with communication, may call attention to itself, and may cause its possessor to be maladjusted (Van Riper, p. 18 1963). Speech intervention is critically needed and will be described, together with listening intervention, in Chapter 6.

Language Problem

We have stated that hard-of-hearing children have listening problems and, in certain instances, speech deficits, both interfering with interpersonal communication, and the former also negatively affecting environmental homeostasis. Complicating these problems is the presence of a third communicative deficit found among hard-of-hearing children—namely, language delay or linguistic deficit. Since unilateral and especially bilateral hearing loss result in less sound input during the formative years of life, beginning in infancy, language learning opportunities are accordingly reduced. Environmental referents ordinarily seen or heard, or concomitant verbal descriptions, or both, become missed or misidentified. In the event of a glass shattering and the uttering of the comment, "A glass fell and broke," for example, either the salient event or the comment may not be detected or recognized, and, thus, they will not be associated for language learning (Berg, 1976, p. 18). One or the other of these two sound stimuli, or both, may be too far off for the hard-of-hearing child to hear, or may be on the impaired-ear side of the head, or may be masked by competing speech or ambient noise.

The language deficit of the entire population of hard-of-hearing children is a very large educational problem. The fact that most hearing loss in childhood is not even recognized, so that remedial steps can be taken, intensifies this very serious problem. Children with unilateral loss as well as youngsters with even slight bilateral impairments are affected. As might be expected, the greater the hearing loss, typically the greater the language deficit. A question arises, however, with respect to the relative impact upon language of certain categories of hearing loss. For example, would a moderate unilateral hearing loss result in a greater language deficit or delay than a marginal (slight) bilateral loss or vice versa?

Large-scale studies need to be conducted among identified hard-of-hearing children in the schools in order to clarify the relationships among categories of hearing loss and extents of language deficits. Such variables as intelligence and socioeconomic background would have to be ruled out or held constant. These and other factors complicate the impact of hearing loss upon language acquisition (Hamilton & Owrid, 1974).

Prior studies relating hearing loss and language deficit have been almost entirely restricted to children with mild or greater bilateral impairment. These studies document that such hard-of-hearing children are delayed or retarded in vocabulary comprehension and that the vocabulary gap increases rather than decreases with age. Using a picture vocabulary test, Young and Mc-Connell (1957) discovered that each of 20 hard-of-hearing children scored lower than an individually-matched normal hearing child. These hard-of-hearing children were 8–14 years of age and had decibel losses of 42–85 in their better ears. Using a picture test of basic concepts, J. Davis (1974) found that 24 hard-of-hearing children fell further and further behind their normal hearing peers in responding correctly as age increased from 6–8 years. Their losses ranged from 25 to 70 dB in the better ear.

The vocabulary deficit of the hard-of-hearing child is often accompanied by a delay in complex syntactical development. Wilcox and Tobin (1974), for example, found that a group of 11 hard-of-hearing children, with a mean age of 10 years and mean hearing loss in the better ear of 61 dB, scored lower than did normal hearing children in using two transformational rules simultaneously. In a similar study, Davis and Blasdell (1975) found that hard-of-hearing children from 6 to 9 years of age, with hearing loss ranging from 35 to 70 dB in the better ears, were behind in the embedding of relative clauses

Table 1-4.
Difference between expected performance and actual
performance of hard-of-hearing children on various subtests of
the Stanford Achievement Test

Hearing Threshold Level (better ear)	Number	IQ	Word Meaning	Paragraph Meaning	Language	Subtest Average
Less than 15dB	59	105.14	−1.04	−0.47	−0.78	−0.73
15–26 dB	37	100.81	−1.40	−.86	−1.16	−1.11
27–40 dB	6	103.50	−3.40	−1.78	−1.95	−2.31
41–55 dB	9	97.89	−3.84	−2.54	−2.93	−3.08
56–70 dB	5	92.40	−2.78	−2.20	−3.52	−2.78
Total group	116	102.56	−1.66	−0.90	−1.30	−1.25

to form complex sentences. In contrast to deaf children, however, hard of hearing children produce the great majority of sentences with correct grammatical structure. In syntactical maturity, the hard-of-hearing child performs like a younger normal hearing youngster.

Dobie & Berlin (1979) recently studied the impact of a simulated slight bilateral hearing loss upon language input. They recorded sample utterances, shaped them so that the signal would be presented at a 40-phon level, displayed the modified speech oscillographically, and then attenuated the samples by 20 dB. Persons then read the attenuated oscillographs to segment and mark the onset of utterances. These oscillographs revealed that there was a potential loss of transitional information and a degradation of very brief utterances and high-frequency segments in the presence of typical signal-to-noise ratios found in today's schools. A child with a 20-dB bilateral loss might lose or sporadically misunderstand morphological markers as well as inflections carrying subtle nuances, such as those occurring in questions.

Earlier, Quigley and Thomure (1968) had studied the impact of varying degrees of hearing loss upon age-equivalent performance in word meaning, paragraph meaning, and language subtests of the Stanford Achievement Test. The subjects were 116 elementary- and secondary-level students of an Illinois school district. The achievement data for each subgroup of hearing loss are shown in Table 1-4. IQ scores of children from the subgroups fell within normal limits. The subtest scores revealed consistent language-age deficits, beginning with hearing threshold levels in the better ear of less than 15 dB (−0.73 years) and increasing through the 41-55 category (−3.08 years). The age ranges for each subgroup were fairly equally distributed to age 15, when a sharp enrollment drop occurred. The authors hypothesize that when hard-of-hearing children reach legal age, they tend to drop out of school, as these data suggest. This hypothesis is supported by the higher percentage of hearing impairment found among delinquent and prison populations than among the general population (Ross, 1982).

One of the interesting findings of the Quigley and Thomure study was that children with a less than 15-dB hearing loss, including even unilateral impairment, were retarded in knowing the meaning of words and paragraphs and in the selection of appropriate language forms from options presented to them. The deficits in these subtest categories were even greater for children with losses from 15 to 26 dB. The subject averages for these 2 groups were -0.73 years and -1.11 years, respectively. These findings are particularly impressive in that the community of people from which these children were drawn was at a higher-than-average socioeconomic level.

An examination of individual children's scores from the foregoing studies does reveal that some hard-of-hearing children perform better than some normally hearing children (Ross, 1982). This is to be expected because the variable of hearing loss, as significant and powerful as it is, can be compensated for by favorable variables such as high intelligence and early and sustained educational intervention. Ordinarily, however, hearing loss seems to be accompanied by factors that intensify, rather than alleviate, the resultant problems. Before discussing these other factors, other features of the language deficit of the hard of hearing will be reviewed briefly.

In addition to vocabulary and complex syntactical deficits, the hard of hearing have problems in understanding and using the figurative language patterns which are common in normal conversation. These patterns include idioms, metaphors, similes, and personification, which are based on or make use of expressions that do not represent the literal or explicit meaning of a word or words. For example, the expressions "Don't shoot off your mouth" and "He's a ball of fire" may not be understood or used, or, once learned, may be quickly replaced among the peer group with other figurative expressions having the same meaning. The hard-of-hearing child has great difficulty "staying with it" or "moving with the flow." (Ross, 1982, p. 31).

Multiple meanings or synonyms also give the hard-of-hearing child a great deal of trouble. The child may learn or be taught a single meaning of a word, or conversely, only one word to express a general concept. In reality, one word such as "over", may mean "above" or "finished" or "across," to mention just three of its meanings. The word "walk" might be overused by the hard-of-hearing child, whereas nuances of meaning such as "creep", "hike", and "march" would be more appropriately used (Ross, 1982).

The language deficit or delay of the hard-of-hearing child has a deleterious impact on the development of listening skills. Even when hard-of-hearing children can detect and discriminate sounds, they may not recognize words or comprehend sentences because they do not know the meaning of words, figurative expressions, or complex language constructions used by the normally hearing at home and in school. The hard-of-hearing child may become lost in many communicative interchanges because of speech recognition and comprehension deficits. Both parents and teachers may be unaware of this language-induced deficit because it is hidden behind a smoke screen of speech comprehension when familiar vocabulary and literal expressions are embedded in less complex sentences, particularly when the hard-of-hearing child can look and listen and a single person is speaking.

Hearing-loss-induced language deficits compound the ordinarily challenging learning-to-read process from preschool and kindergarten through high school. During the readiness period of preschool and kindergarten, the hard-of-hearing child may lack the language facility to share experiences with others. At the first through third grade levels, the child may be slow in learning a sight vocabulary or in acquiring a phonetic ability to sound out new words. Grades four through six are even more trying times for the hard-of-hearing child. By this time, children are expected to have developed basic reading skills and therefore are exposed to a tremendous increase in printed words, expressions, and syntactical forms. Unfortunately, the hard-of-hearing child does not have sufficient spoken referents for this more advanced reading material. The problem is further compounded during grades seven through twelve, the refinement period of reading, with the hard-of-hearing child falling further and further behind normal hearing peers (Pauls, 1958).

The spoken language and reading deficits of the hard-of-hearing child tend to affect corresponding writing activities in school. Compositions may be limited to fewer words and to less complex and more literal written expressions than are those of normal hearing students. There may be a lack of generative, creative, and expansive forms with a corresponding dearth of ideas and originality.

Cognition and Academic Deficit

Sensory and communicative deficits affect the cognitive maturation of hard-of-hearing children. Cognition may be defined as personal knowledge of the world (Boothroyd, 1982, p. 29). During the early years of life, sense organs are stimulated and neural patterns generated so that a basic level of cognition is established. Using Piagetian test tasks of basic thinking and reasoning, Furth (1971) discovered that even deaf children seem to perform on par with their normally hearing peers. Levine (1976), however, states that the actual cognitive competence of children is depressed to a greater or lesser degree as a result of linguistic, experiential, and communicative deficiencies.

Boothroyd (1982, p. 29) indicates that cognition and language are interdependent. Before language can develop, a basic level of cognition must exist, and yet language promotes the maturation of cognition. Furthermore, listening and speaking and other activities modify the sensory experiences and knowledge of the world that a child ordinarily has. A hierarchical organization and reorganization of sensory experiences takes place as more and more sensory experiences occur. With sufficient sensory input and communicative skills, the child's cognition or model of the world develops to become increasingly complex.

Four stages of cognitive-linguistic development may be outlined in the development of a person's world model. During the first stage, children become increasingly aware of qualities, patterns, similarities, differences, and correspondences. Depending upon hearing, they also begin to associate their own speech movements with sounds of speech in their environments. By three or four months of age, children ordinarily move into the second stage of cognitive-linguistic development. This is a time of rapid perceptual and motor development and motor exploration and the discovery that speech sounds can manipulate people. Categories become part of cognition and sensory impressions are placed in them. Verbal labels, or symbols, are learned as referents for objects, feelings, and events. By 18–24 months, children usually enter the third stage of cognitive-linguistic development. At this point, new categories are created to process the expanding perceptual input. Verbal labels take on new and more abstract meanings or are combined into sentences. The final stage of cognitive-linguistic development coincides with the beginning of formal schooling. The child is expected to have sufficient mastery of language and an abstract enough world model to learn to read and write and converse with others (Boothroyd, 1982, pp. 32–35).

To the extent that a child is shut out from auditory input, that child's cognition may not mature. The listening, speech, and, particularly, language deficits of the hard-of-hearing child will impede advanced cognitive development. The greater the hearing loss, the more affected the communication and the more limited the cognitive-linguistic development. Restricted language content (vocabulary and semantics), form (syntax), and use (pragmatics) associated with unilateral and especially bilateral hearing loss will curtail the child's world model, or internal description of reality. The hard-of-hearing child will appear as a less sophisticated or less verbally knowledgeable individual than the typical normally hearing child.

The verbal-cognitive deficits of hard-of-hearing children are accompanied by reduced scores on tests of academic achievement. For example, an early study of 100 children attending school in Kentucky with an average 50-dB hearing loss in the better ears revealed a mean academic deficit of 2.24 years. These children, aged 7–17, repeated 57 grades (Kodman, 1963). Other, more recent, studies have shown highly similar results (Paul & Young, 1975; Quigley & Thomure, 1968).

Verbal-cognitive academic deficits are directly related to degree of hearing impairment. Using a 6871-person national sample of hearing-impaired children and youth in special educational settings, Jensema (1975) found that scores on mathematical concepts and computation and, especially, vocabulary and reading comprehension were depressed increasingly as bilateral hearing loss increased from mild to profound. In Boatner's (1965) and McClure's (1966) earlier surveys in schools and classes for the deaf, most children 16 years or older read at grade level 5.3 or lower, or were at least 5 years retarded in verbal-cognitive development.

The direct relationship between hearing loss and achievement deficits also exists among children in regular educational settings. For example, in the Quigley and Thomure study reported earlier, academic subtest deficits averaged three-quarters of one year for children with marginal unilateral and bilateral hearing loss and increased to 3 years for children with moderate bilateral hearing impairment.

The linguistic, cognitive, and academic deficits of hard-of-hearing children are usually based in sensory rather than intellectual deficiencies. When the nonverbal or performance portions of intelligence tests are individually administered to such children, they score comparatively well. As an example, the author recalls an 18-year-old university student with a moderate bilateral loss. She had scored 123 on the performance portion of the Wechsler Adult Intelligence Scale but only 73 on the verbal battery (Berg, 1976, p. 26).

The academic gap between the hard-of-hearing student and the normal hearing student characteristically increases with age. A one-year retardation in the fourth grade, for example, might become a 2-year deficit in the eighth grade, and a 3-year gap in the twelfth grade. Often, hard-of-hearing students completing high school require extensive remedial assistance before they can succeed in technical or professional post-secondary study programs; these same students become better prospects for vocational training, which requires less time involvement and much less academic background.

Emotional and Social Problems

Hard-of-hearing children understandably also have a higher-than-normal incidence of emotional and social problems. There is a characteristic restriction on personality, but no indication of mental illness (Myklebust, 1960, pp. 46–48). The hearing loss and associated deficits seem to magnify normally unfavorable emotional and social tendencies in children (Wright, 1970).

Social problems appear to be more prevalent in children with mild or moderate bilateral hearing loss than in those with severe impairments (ASHA, 1983), with girls being recognized as showing more marked differences in amount and pattern of maladjusted behavior than do boys (Fisher, 1966). In an Illinois school district, 121 children were identified as having bilateral hearing loss in excess of 40 dB. Their teachers rated only 11 of the 121 as normally participating class members. Twenty-eight were rated as socially introverted and 17 were considered social problems (Bothwell, 1967).

As a group, hard-of-hearing children seem to be less well accepted than are their normal hearing peers. Elser (1959) studied the social position of children aged 9–12 from several elementary schools in rural Tennessee who had bilateral hearing loss exceeding 45 dB. Generally, the hard of hearing scored relatively low in friendship and reputation.

The social problems of the hard-of-hearing are reciprocally related to emotional problems (Boothroyd, 1982, p. 37). With moderate or severe bilateral loss, children often feel isolated, inadequate, and helpless. They may become bitter and resentful, or depressed and apathetic, or more on guard than usual (Wright, 1970). They become masters of the neutral response: smiling, saying yes, and periodically nodding their heads affirmatively, while unaware of what others are communicating. The hard of hearing may either keep quiet or try to dominate conversation to avoid having to understand what is unclear (Vernon, 1970).

Negative feelings and corresponding inappropriate reactions are also associated with unilateral hearing impairment. A person may miss a remark that others hear and become annoyed, confused, or embarrassed (Giolas & Wark, 1967). This occurs often when the talker is located on the side of the poor ear or when there is background noise in the listening environment (Giolas, 1982). Speech misunderstandings can lead to withdrawal, acting out, talking too much, or other undesirable compensatory reactions characteristic of many individuals with bilateral hearing loss.

The Vineland Social Maturity scale, which was developed to assess mentally retarded persons, clarifies the social problems of those who are hard-of-hearing. Social maturity is defined as competence in caring for oneself and assisting with the care of others. Three levels of social competence are outlined: self-help, self-direction, and care of others. Normal age guidelines for self-help, self-direction, and care of others are 7–8, 18, and 25 years of age, respectively. Hard-of-hearing children ordinarily develop self-help skills, such as feeding and dressing themselves, on schedule but fall behind in self-direction competencies such as using the telepone or going out on their own. They tend to fall still further behind in caring for others, being slower in learning to provide for the future and to contribute to the general welfare of society. When the hard-of-hearing person achieves social maturity, it is ordinarily at an older age than that of an individual with normal hearing (Doll, 1953; Myklebust, 1960, p. 214).

Social and emotional problems of older hard-of-hearing children and youth may be uncovered when using a self-report scale such as the Hearing Performance Inventory described by Giolas (1982). Clients are asked to read a series of 90 items and to rate themselves. A 5-point scale provides 5 response options for each item: practically always; frequently; about half the time; occasionally; and, almost never. A sample item appears below:

> You are talking with five or six friends. When you miss something that was said, do you ask the person talking to repeat it?

This particular item falls into the category of response to auditory failure. Other categories of response include understanding speech, intensity of sound, and social, personal, and occupational situations.

The Hearing Performance Inventory has been designed to provide a systematic procedure for identifying the scope of problem areas resulting from hearing impairment and accompanying listening deficiencies. A major problem with such an inventory, however, is that people tend not to reveal their true perceptions when they perform undesirably in life situations. Giolas (1982) states that the reality of perceptions to the inventory items and the degree to which they manifest a handicap is unknown. A person administering the inventory may note a significant difference between the client's response to items and response to actual situations similar in nature to these items.

Parents, Teachers, and Society

The problems of hard-of-hearing children are often compounded further by undesirable reactions from parents, teachers, and society at large. Prior to the identification and diagnosis of hearing loss, there is general misunderstanding of the characteristics and needs of these chidlren. In the regular schools, for example, the unidentified hard-of-hearing child may be labeled as uncooperative, mentally defective, or emotionally disturbed (O'Neill, 1964, p. 107). Once parents find out that their child has a hearing loss, they may enter a state of denial, confusion, and general ineffectiveness. Some parents may even categorize their child as deaf, reduce language stimulation, and withdraw communicative and social interaction (Ross & Calvert, 1967). The complex nature of hearing and various ramifications of hearing loss in childhood escape the understanding of even professionals who could offer helpful guidance to parents, teachers, and other key educational facilitators. Boothroyd (1982) states that a typical withdrawal of interaction by the parents will be repeated by society at large. There is definitely a period of adjustment and learning that both parents and society require before they can be expected to positively influence the lives of hard-of-hearing children. A vicious cycle can occur in which hearing loss and associated secondary impairments (e.g., listening and emotional problems) trigger negative parental and societal reactions, which in turn causes the child to have further educational and social problems. Each time this cycle repeats itself, it can result in further deterioration of the child's emotional well-being and educational adjustment.

Often, parents, teachers, and others do not conceptualize the characteristics and needs of hard-of-hearing children, even when they no longer deny the hearing loss and no longer withdraw from the child. They may not, furthermore, be committed to providing or able to provide the informed, systematic, and sustained special assistance needed to compensate for unilateral and particularly bilateral hearing loss in childhood. Currently, sufficient appropriate professional assistance is not available throughout the country to alleviate this lack of conceptualization and commitment or ability exhibited by so many people who interact so often with hard-of-hearing children (Blair & Berg, 1982). "Man's struggle toward enlightenment is slow, faltering, and in many instances, haphazard" (Silverman, 1978).

Vocational Problems

The deficiencies of hard-of-hearing children already described—particularly communicative, cognitive, emotional, and social deficits—can have a severe to devastating impact upon a person's preparing for suitable employment, finding the right job, and advancing vocationally. The importance of one's employment to one's well-being is ably described by Kevin Marshall (1982):

> In Western society, probably no other single elective variable influences a person as comprehensively as the choice of work. Employment, as the primary determinant of a person's economic situation and subsequent standard of living, is a major social discriminator. It determines the type of activity and environment the person will be immersed in for nearly one third of his or her life, and is a predominant factor in making the majority of daily life decisions, such as when to eat, sleep, take vacations, and the like. Psychologically, the type, level of remuneration, and physical setting of the employment determine which social values are ascribed to different jobs. Subsequently, the job often becomes a yardstick by which many persons measure the worth of themselves and others.
>
> Common personal variables of the hard of hearing detrimental to competitive job search, placement, and retention are basic hearing limitations, communication problems, educational deficit, lack of "real world" experiences, and feelings of exclusion from other employees and the employer (Marshall, 1982). As a result, a disproportionately large percentage of hard-of-hearing children, when they become adults, become vocationally disadvantaged, being relegated to lower socioeconomic positions in our society than their potential and efforts warrant.

SUMMARY

In this chapter, a foundation has been laid for the remaining chapters of the book by detailing the characteristics of the target population. The many interacting deficiencies of hard-of-hearing students have been detailed. The point has been made that any degree of hearing loss puts a student at educational risk. The basic listening problem of the target population, introduced in Chapter 1, should be kept in mind while reading the entire book. Chapters 6 and 7 will provide further information on this basic problem and how its effects can be alleviated.

REFERENCES

American Speech-Language-Hearing Association. Audiology services in the schools position statement. *ASHA*, 1983, *25*, 53–60.
Berg F. The Locus of the education of the hard of hearing child. In F Berg & S Fletcher (Eds.),

The hard of hearing child: Clinical and educational management. New York: Grune & Stratton, 1970, pp. 13–26.

Berg F. *Educational audiology: Hearing and speech management.* New York: Grune & Stratton, 1976.

Berg F. Listening Handbook. Precision programs for the Hearing Impaired. Part 1 of the Listening and Speech package (LAS-PAC). New York: Grune & Stratton, 1978.

Bess F. Children with unilateral hearing loss. *Journal of the Academy of Rehabilitative Audiology.* 1982, 15, 131–144.

Black J. Speech pathology for the deaf. In L Conner (Ed.) *Speech for the deaf child: Knowledge and use.* Washington, D.C.: The Alexander Graham Bell Association for the Deaf, 1971, pp. 154–169.

Blair J & Berg F. Problems and needs of Hard-of-Hearing Students and a Model for the Delivery of Services to the Schools. ASHA, 1982, 8, 541–546.

Boatner E. The need of a realistic approach to the education of the deaf. Presented to the Joint Convention of the California Association of Parents of Deaf and Hard-of-Hearing Children, California Association of Teachers of Deaf and Hard of Hearing, the California Association of the Deaf, Los Angeles, November 6, 1965.

Boothroyd A. *Hearing impairments in young children.* Englewood Cliffs, New Jersey: Prentice-Hall, 1982.

Bothwell H. *Developing a comprehensive program for hearing impaired children on a state-wide basis.* Proceedings of Office of Education sponsored Institute on Characteristics and Needs of the Hard-of-Hearing Child. Unpublished material, Utah State University, 1967.

Byers V. Initial consonant intelligibility by hearing-impaired children. *Journal of Speech and Hearing Research,* 1973, *16,* 48–55.

Davis H. Abnormal hearing and deafness. In H Davis & S R Silverman (Eds.), *Hearing and Deafness.* New York: Holt, Rinehart and Winston, 1978, pp. 87–146, 270–274.

Davis J. Performance of young hearing-impaired children on a test of basic concepts. *Journal of Speech and Hearing Research,* 1974, *17,* 342–351.

Davis J & Blasdell R. Perceptual strategies employed by normal-hearing and hearing-impaired children in the comprehension of sentences containing relative clauses. *Journal of Speech and Hearing Research,* 1975, *18,* 281–295.

Denes & Pinson E. *The Speech Chain.* New Jersey: Bell Telephone Laboratories, 1963.

Dobie R & Berlin C. Influence of otitis media on hearing and development. *Annals of Otology, Rhinology, and Laryngology,* 1979, 88, Supplement 60, 48–53.

DiCarlo L. Speech, language, and cognitive abilities of the hard of hearing. *Proceedings of the Institute on Aural Rehabilitation,* SRS 212-T-68. Denver: University of Denver, 1968, 45–66.

Doll E. The measurement of social competence. Minneapolis: Educational Test Bureau, 1953.

Downs M. Contributions of mild hearing loss to auditory language learning problems. In R Roeser & M Downs (Eds.). *Auditory Disorders in School children.* New York: Thieme-Stratton, pp. 177–189.

Eisenson J & Ogilvie M. Communication disorders in children. New York: McMillan, 1983 pp. 161–162

Elser R. The social position of hearing handicapped children the regular grades. *Exceptional Child,* 1959, *25,* 305–309.

Erber N. Speech correction through the use of acoustic models. In J Subtelny (Ed.), *Speech assessment and speech improvement for the hearing impaired.* Washington, D.C.: The Alexander Graham Bell Association for the Deaf, 1980, pp. 222–241.

Erber N. *Auditory training.* Washington, D.C.: The Alexander Graham Bell Association for the Deaf, 1982. pp. 21–24.

Feistritzer E. Commentary by the publisher. Washington, D.C.: Feistritzer Publications, *Department of Education Weekly,* July 18, 1983. p. 7.

Fellendorf G. *An EDUHEALTH delivery service index: A profile of education and health services to young hearing impaired children and their parents.* Washington, D.C.: Alexander Graham Bell Association for the Deaf, 1975, p. 11.

Fisher B. The social and emotional adjustment of children with impaired hearing attending ordinary classes. *British Journal of Educational Psychology,* 1966, *36,* 319–321.

Fletcher S. Introduction, In F Berg & S Fletcher (Eds.), *The hard of hearing child: Clinical and educational management.* New York: Grune & Stratton, 1970, pp. 3–6.

Furth H. Linguistic deficiency and thinking: Research with deaf subjects 1964–69. *Psychological Bulletin,* 1971, *76,* 58–72.

Giolas T. *Hearing-handicapped adults.* Englewood Cliffs, New Jersey: Prentice-Hall, 1982.

Giolas T & Wark D. Communication problems associated with unilateral hearing loss. *Journal of Speech and Hearing Disorders.* 1967, *41,* 336–343.

Hamilton P & Owrid H. Comparisons of hearing impairment and socio-cultural disadvantage in relation to verbal retardation. *British Journal of Audiology,* 1974, *8,* 27–32.

Jensema C. *The relationship between academic achievement and the demographic characteristics of hearing impaired children and youth.* Office of Demographic Studies, Washington, D.C. Gallaudet College, Series R, No. 2, 1975.

Kodman F. Education status of hard of hearing children in the classroom. *Journal of Speech and Hearing Disorders,* 1963, *28,* 297–299.

Levine E. Psychological contribution. In R Frisina (Ed.), *A Bicentennial monograph on hearing impairment: Trends in the USA.* Washington, D.C.; The Alexander Graham Bell Association for the Deaf, 1976, pp. 23–33.

Ling D. *Speech and the hearing impaired child.* Washington, D.C.: The Alexander Graham Bell Association for the Deaf, 1976.

Ling D. *The detection factor.* Montreal: McGill University, 1981. (Videocassette)

Marshall K. The vocational impact of hearing impairment as viewed by the vocational rehabilitation counselor. In R. Hull (Ed.) *Rehabilitative Audiology.* New York: Grune & Stratton, 1982, 161–169.

McClure W. Current problems and trends in the education of the deaf. *Deaf American,* 1966, *31,* 8–14.

Myklebust H. *The psychology of deafness: Sensory deprivation, learning, and adjustment.* New York: Grune & Stratton, 1960, pp. 46–48.

Newby H. *Audiology.* Englewood Cliffs, New Jersey: Prentice-Hall, 1979, p. 62.

Nickerson R. Characteristics of the speech of deaf persons. *Volta Review,* 1975, *77,* 342–362.

O'Neill J. *The hard of hearing.* Englewood Cliffs, New Jersey: Prentice-Hall, 1964 p. 107.

Paul R & Young B. *The child with a mild sensorineural hearing loss: The failure Syndrome.* Paper delivered at the International Congress on Education of the Deaf, Tokyo, 1975.

Pauls M. Language development through reading. *Volta Review,* 1958, *60,* 105–107; 142.

Quigley S & Thomure F. *Some effects of hearing impairment upon school performance.* Springfield, Illinois: Division of Special Education Services, 1968.

Richardson M & Donaldson J. Middle ear fluid. *American Family Physician.* June 1981, *23,* 159–163.

Risberg A, Agelfors E, & Boberg F. Measurements of frequency-discrimination ability of severely and profoundly hearing impaired children. *Speech Transmission Laboratory QPSR 2–3.* Stockholm: Royal Institute of Technology, 1975, 40–48.

Ross M. *Hard of hearing children in regular schools.* Englewood Cliffs, New Jersey: Prentice-Hall, 1982, pp. 3–4.

Ross M & Calvert. The semantics of deafness. *Volta Review,* 1967, 69, 644–649.

Ross M, & Lerman J. A picture identification test for hearing impaired children. *Journal of Speech and Hearing Research,* 1970, *13,* 17, 23, 44–53.

Rupp R & Stockdell K. The roles of speech protocols in audiolody. In R. Rupp & K. Stockdell (Eds.) *Speech protocols in Audiology.* New York: Grune & Stratton, 1980, pp. 5–38, p. 23.

Sanders D. *Aural rehabilitation: A management model.* Englewood Cliffs, New Jersey: Prentice-Hall, 1982.

Sanders E. When are speech sounds learned? *Journal of Speech and Hearing Disorders,* 1972, *37,* 26–29, 55–63.

Silverman SR. From Aristotle to Bell and beyond. In H Davis & SR Silverman (Eds.), *Hearing and Deafness.* New York: Holt, Rinehart and Winston, 1978, 421–432.

Trybus R. National data on rated speech intelligibility of hearing-impaired children. In J Subtleny (Ed.) *Speech assessment and speech improvement for the hearing impaired.* Washington, D.C.: The Alexander Graham Bell Association for the Deaf, 1980, pp. 67–71.

Van Riper C. *Speech correction: Principles and methods.* Englewood Cliffs; New Jersey: Prentice-Hall, 1963, p. 18.

Vernon M. The psychological examination. In F Berg & S Fletcher (Eds). *The hard of hearing child: Clinical and educational management.* New York: Grune & Stratton, 1970, pp. 217–231.

Wedenberg E. Auditory training in historical perspective. In F Bess, B Freeman, & S Sinclair (Eds.), *Amplification in education.* Washington, D.C.: Alexander Graham Bell Association for the Deaf, 1981, pp. 1–25.

West J & Weber J. Phonological analysis of the spontaneous language of a four-year-old, hard-of-hearing child. *Journal of Speech and Hearing Disorders,* 1973, *38,* 25–35.

Wilcox J & Tobin, H. Linguistic performance of hard of hearing and normal hearing children. *Journal of Speech and Hearing Research,* 1974, *17,* 286–293.

Wright W. Counseling. In F Berg & S Fletcher (Eds.), *The hard of hearing child: Clinical and educational management.* New York: Gruen & Stratton, 1970, pp. 155–174.

Young D & McConnel F. Retardation of vocabulary development in hard of hearing children. *Exceptional Child,* 1957, *23,* 368–370.

James C. Blair

2
Services Needed

Blair and Berg (1982) described a model for the delivery of services to the hearing-impaired in the regular schools. This model was developed in an attempt to meet the identified needs of hearing-impaired children. This identification was derived initially from the literature and then from a Delphi analysis (Dalkey, 1969) and a Fault Tree analysis (Witkin & Stephens, 1973). Through the use of these various procedures, 5 competencies were identified as those essential for a professional attempting to provide appropriate services to the hearing impaired; the professional must be able to: (1) Obtain, integrate, and synthesize diagnostic information; (2) Obtain additional educational and audiological test results; (3) Evaluate the available environmental and educational resources; (4) Plan appropriate programs; and, (5) Implement these programs.

This chapter will highlight methods by which these five tasks may be achieved. The model proposed by Blair and Berg (1982) and subsequently modified by Wilson-Vlotman (1984) will be used as the framework for discussion. This proposed model will then be contrasted with what is actually being done in the schools, as described by Wilson-Vlotman (1984). Finally, the problems associated with trying to increase and improve services to the hearing impaired will be discussed.

THE DELIVERY OF SERVICES MODEL

Before the hearing-impaired child can receive appropriate services, it is critical that such a youngster be identified. As suggested by Roeser and Northern (1981), only the children with obvious hearing loss tend to be

25

identified. A comprehensive screening program thus needs to be in place in the schools so that all children with educationally significant hearing loss can be identified. Wilson-Vlotman (1984) found in her nationwide study that most states have some kind of identification/screening program. Identification programs, however, need to be followed by comprehensive audiological follow-up. It is not sufficient to identify youngsters with hearing loss; there must be appropriate follow-up services provided. Chapter 4 describes appropriate audiological assessment in the schools and amplifies the way in which the information obtained from the audiologic evaluation can enhance the delivery of services to the hearing impaired. It is also important that data from audiologic evaluations be correlated with findings from otologic examinations and from special auditory test results when auditory problems are suspected. Once diagnostic audiologic and otologic evaluations are completed, there is a need for a complete psycho-educational assessment. It is only when a complete picture of the hearing-impaired child is obtained that an appropriate intervention strategy can be formulated. Too often, it is assumed that problems of hearing-impaired individuals are limited to hearing loss only. There is ample evidence to suggest that hearing-impaired children fall consistently below their hearing peers academically (Blair, Peterson, & Viehweg, 1985; Davis, 1974; Davis, Shepard, Stelmachowicz & Gorga, 1981; Quigley & Thomure, 1978). The hard-of-hearing child also often evidences symptoms of emotional and/or social immaturity (Levine, 1960; Schlesinger & Meadow; 1972). The hearing impaired also have a higher incidence of visual problems than do the normal hearing (Allen, 1980; Mohindra, 1976; Myklebust, 1960; Pollard & Neumaier, 1974). There is also some research suggesting that motor problems are more prevalent among the hearing impaired than among the general population (Myklebust, 1960). The need for a *complete* assessment of the hearing-impaired child is therefore very important.

As Shepard, Davis, Gorga, & Stelmachowicz (1981) discovered, appropriate assessment information is frequently not present in the files of hearing-impaired students. If appropriate habilitational programs are to be provided, complete information about each individual must be collected. The psycho-educational evaluation is described in Chapter 3.

In conjunction with the above evaluative procedures, there is a critical need for the appropriate use of amplification. Blair (1977), Bess and McConnel (1981), Gaeth and Lounsbury (1966), Matkin (1984), Nault (1983), Roeser and Downs (1981), and Ross (1982), to name but a few, all describe the need for appropriate fitting and careful monitoring of the amplification systems of hearing-impaired youngsters. In spite of this, it appears that there is still a serious problem in the monitoring of hearing aids in the regular schools. Wilson-Vlotman (1984) asked 225 educational audiologists who work full-time in the schools the question: "Who monitors the hard-of-hearing child's hearing aid?" The response to this question revealed that only 10 percent of the educational audiologists monitor the aids themselves (Table 2-1) and that

Table 2-1.
Individuals who have primary responsibility for monitoring
hearing aids on a daily basis, as perceived by educational
audiologists

Individual Monitoring	Percentage Reporting
Teacher of the deaf	58%
Regular classroom teacher	14%
Educational audiologist	10%
Parents	6%
Speech-language pathologist	4%
Students	2%
No one	2%
Other	4%

From Wilson-Vlotman, A. Practices and perceptions of educational audiology in the United
States. Unpublished doctoral dissertation, Utah State University, 1984. With permission.

a variety of other professionals (at least so it was perceived) monitor the aids
more regularly. One of the startling findings of the Wilson-Vlotman study was
that 73 percent of the educational audiologists perceived that either teachers
of the deaf or regular classroom teachers monitored the hearing aid. Many
teachers of the deaf and most regular classroom teachers do not know how
to troubleshoot hearing aids, however (Jones, 1982). Another significant
group which was expected to monitor the aids was parents; however, Blair,
Wright, and Pollard (1981) found that parents have very limited information
about their child's hearing aid or their child's hearing loss, in spite of many
years of audiological testing and information. Chapter 5 will address amplification considerations for hearing-impaired youngsters.

Once the hearing-impaired youngster has been fitted with an appropriate
amplification system and once an appropriate evaluation has been completed,
the educational program needs to be implemented. Clark and Watkins (1985),
Lillie and Trohanis (1976), Watkins (1984), and others have discussed the
value of parental involvement in the habilitational/educational process. As
children move into public education, however, the parents seem to be rapidly
excluded from active participation in the educational process. It is of utmost
importance that parents participate in the educational process with their
hearing-impaired children through at least middle school or junior high
school. Gradual withdrawal from the process needs to occur during or after
junior high school so that the adolescent hearing-impaired individual can
achieve a level of independence. The roles of parents and parental issues will
be discussed in Chapter 8.

Another aspect of the educational program relates to the role administrators play in the education of the youngster with a hearing loss. Unfortunately, many educational audiologists view administrators in the same way as
does the person who said ". . . the greatest stumbling block to education that

we face . . . is administrators" (Berg & Blair, 1980). This negative view of administrators must be changed if there is to be an alteration in the amount and type of services provided to the hearing impaired in the regular schools. The only viable way to make changes in the educational system is through administrators. In Chapter 8, administrative issues will be discussed.

Still another aspect of appropriate intervention relates to the selection of teachers and classrooms to maximize the learning environment of the hearing-impaired student. There is an increasing body of information which highlights the need for better acoustic treatment of classrooms (Finitzo-Hieber, 1981; Finitzo-Hieber & Tillman, 1978; Ross & Giolas, 1978). The literature suggests that noise and/or reverberation will have a negative influence on the listening ability of most hard-of-hearing youngsters. Chapter 7 addresses the acoustic needs of hearing-impaired children in regular schools. It is obvious that teachers have a significant effect on the learning of children. Ross (1978) suggests that an effective teacher will facilitate the cognitive growth of children even in a poor learning environment. If an appropriate environment is provided along with an effective teacher, however, the educational benefits will be even more significant. In Chapter 8, the role of teachers will be discussed in detail.

Once all of the above have been achieved, many hard-of-hearing youngsters are going to need individual attention in the areas of speech, listening, language, and reading. Jones (1982) studied the views of a variety of professionals serving the hearing impaired in the regular schools. She surveyed speech-language pathologists, regular classroom teachers serving hard-of-hearing children, administrators, and educational audiologists. Jones found that perceptions regarding who should provide services to the hearing impaired depended upon the individual asked. One of the findings in the Jones study, however, was that no professional working in the regular school views the total educational management of the hard of hearing as his or her primary responsibility. It becomes increasingly clear that we, as a profession, are failing to provide comprehensive services to hard-of-hearing individuals. Chapters 6 and 8 will address comprehensive case management concepts.

DIFFERENT MODELS OF DELIVERY

A variety of conceptual models of delivery of service to the hearing impaired have been proposed (ASHA, 1980; Berg, 1976; Blair & Berg, 1982; Ross & Calvert, 1977). These various models take different forms and can be described using the schema proposed by the Ad Hoc Committee on Extension of Audiological Services in the Schools (ASHA, 1980). This committee identified 4 models of delivery of audiological services presently used in the field, Yater (1978) described a fifth model.

The first model is described as a parent referral model. In this model,

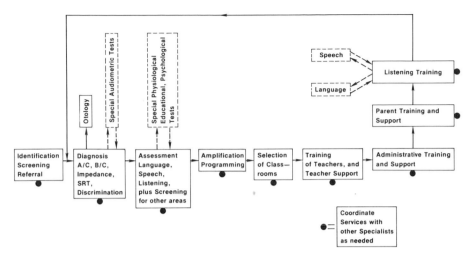

Fig. 2-1. Delivery of services by the educational audiologist. The solid lines indicate that the educational audiologist will be directly involved with these activities. The dotted lines suggest that the educational audiologist may be involved either directly or indirectly with these services.

identification services are provided by the local education authority (LEA). The parents or primary caregivers then have the responsibility to arrange for further evaluation at local medical and audiological facilities. Parents/caregivers are then expected to report the results and recommendations to the LEA, which initiates intervention procedures. The model is low-cost and low-control, and has low information flow between all parties concerned. In addition, the school is responsible for few of the necessary service provisions. Compliance with federal law is difficult to determine due to the involvement of outside services. Also, because there are generally no professionals in the LEA who fully understand the need for comprehensive services, the parents are left to tell the LEA what services need to be provided and to explain the educational problems that their children may have. Obviously, in this model, a great many of the educational needs of hearing-impaired children are overlooked.

A second model is a school-based or self-contained delivery service. In this model, all necessary services are provided by the LEA. The audiologist, according to the ASHA Ad Hoc Committee, is responsible for assessment, referral, intervention, coordination, follow-up, and staff development and acts as a member of an interdisciplinary team serving the child. This model comes closest to the one advocated in this book. Generally, compliance with the law is more likely in this model, since execution of the program is under the direct control of the educational agency. The cost of the model is, however, high due to the salaries and equipment which the agency must provide.

A third model is a school- and community-based model. Under this model, both the community and the school share in the responsibility of providing services. Clinical assessment is usually completed outside the LEA, with the school audiologist interpreting the information for the school. The LEA has in this model, a great degree of control over services and information flow. The costs, however, remain high under this arrangement. Compliance with the law will vary with the ability of the audiologist to elicit cooperation from service providers.

A fourth model is a contractual agreement model. Under this arrangement, the LEA contracts with community service agencies to provide for audiological services. The degree and nature of the contracts may vary, but the school system retains the responsibility for ensuring comprehensive services. Compliance with the law is accomplished when an appropriate contract is drawn and followed. The costs incurred in this model will vary according to the level of services required.

A fifth model has been described by Yater (1978). While it fits within the third model described above, it contains some unique elements. Under this arrangement, the school audiologist makes referrals to community services for audiological assessment and the school audiologist provides the interpretation of the data. The audiologist also serves as a "hearing clinician", providing direct tutorial help to hearing-impaired children in academic areas of concern. The audiologist thus serves much as an itinerant teacher of the hearing impaired. These models illustrate the 5 general methods currently employed for providing audiological services in the schools, and, to a great extent, dictate the role functions the educational audiologist undertakes.

The authors of this book maintain that a more complete, and, indeed, appropriate model for meeting the needs of the hearing impaired in regular schools is that proposed in this book and illustrated in Figure 2-1. Regardless of the theoretical position one takes, it is important that some consensus be reached concerning the kinds of services that the hearing impaired are to have available to them in the regular schools. As suggested above, the literature addresses the need for a comprehensive management program. Given this need, the study completed by Wilson-Vlotman (1984) is enlighting concerning the kinds of services currently provided to the hearing impaired in the United States.

SERVICES PROVIDED BY EDUCATIONAL AUDIOLOGISTS

Wilson-Vlotman (1984) sent a questionnaire to 225 educational audiologists in each of the 48 continental United States. She received responses from 203 (92 percent) of these individuals. One of the questions related to the way in which educational audiologists spend their time. Table 2-2 illustrates the way in which individuals responded to the question: "What per-

Table 2-2.
Time allocation of the average educational audiologist in the
United States

Tasks	Percentage of Time
Diagnostics	
Identification audiometry, screening	9%
Audiological assessment (diagnostic audiometry)	37%
Central auditory assessment	2%
Classroom management	
Hearing aids, FM systems, etc. (monitoring & maintaining)	12%
Earmolds (fitting, cleaning, repairing)	3%
Indirect services	
Consultation (teachers, parents, administrators)	9%
Counseling (parents, teachers, students)	6%
Direct child services	
Tutoring, aural rehabilitation	7%
Educational assessment	1%
Leadership	
Administration	9%
Supervision (students in training, services)	4%
Research	.6%
Other	.4%

From Wilson-Vlotman A. Practices and perceptions of educational audiology in the United States. Unpublished doctoral dissertation, Utah State University, 1984. With permission.

centage of *time* do you spend each month in the following activities?" Table 1-2 details the 13 categories to which respondents could react and indicates the educational audiologists' average responses.

Notice that educational audiologists reported spending 63 percent of their time, on the average, in performing some form of assessment or providing repair or troubleshooting services. Another 13 percent of their time is used in supervision or administration. Educational audiologists spend 8 percent of their time providing direct services to the hearing impaired in the regular schools. The vast majority of available time is evidently used for some form of diagnostic service, while very little time is spent with students, teachers, parents, or administrators. This allocation of time might be appropriate if there are other professionals in the system who are providing comprehensive services to the hearing impaired.

Discrepancies in Service

If the model presented in Figure 2-1 is considered as encompassing the spectrum of services necessary for the hearing impaired, then the task is to identify services which are currently being provided and those which still need to be provided to discover any discrepancies between what *is* and what *ought to be*. Given the data in the Wilson-Vlotman (1984) study, it is possible to outline with some confidence a typical month for an educational audiologist. Given an average month of 22 working days, and taking as an average day 8 hours, the following appears to be the amount of time spent in various activities: 11 days each month are spent in providing diagnostic evaluation and assessment services; three days are spent providing indirect services; another 3 days are spent keeping hearing aids and audiological equipment in repair; 3 days are spent on various administrative tasks such as writing reports, staffings, IEP meetings, and similar activities; and 2 days are spent working directly with students providing services such as auditory training or academic tutoring.

Given this average use of time, what concerns might be raised concerning the delivery of services? The major concern involves hearing aid management. Jones (1982) found that regular classroom teachers, who are expected to monitor the aids, have no knowledge of hearing aids. Teachers of the deaf, traditionally, are not trained to work with hearing aids and generally feel that the aids should be maintained by someone else, preferably an audiologist. Speech-language pathologists also do not view themselves as capable of dealing with hearing aids and usually suggest that audiologists should be responsible for this maintenance. It would seem then, that one of the most important tasks facing an educational audiologist is the care and maintenance of amplification devices. The educational audiologist, it appears, must take primary responsibility for the care and maintenance of hearing aids. Even though the day-to-day monitoring may fall to someone besides the audiologist, it is critical that this professional take the lead in this area for training in the proper use and care of a hearing aid and for constant follow-up. At the moment, this does not appear to be happening.

Another area of concern is the appropriate educational assessment of hard-of-hearing children in order to obtain appropriate educational intervention (Matkin, Hook, & Hixson, 1979). Davis et al. clearly indicate that this is not happening in the schools. The educational audiologist does not view psycho-educational assessment as a primary area of concern. The child with a hearing loss in the schools needs, however, someone to take the lead in managing all aspects of appropriate education. If the educational audiologist does not oversee the program for the hearing impaired, it is clear that no one else will.

Another discrepancy in services needed and services provided involves parents and teachers. The findings of Wilson-Vlotman (1984) suggest that the average educational audiologist has a caseload which is very large, or else has no caseload at all per se; the audiologist is simply expected to serve all the audiological needs of a very large area and a large number of children. Given that the only time remaining for contact with parents and teachers is very small (1–2 hours each week), it is clear that the amount of time available to meet with individual teachers or parents is extremely limited. The ability of the educational audiologist to properly manage the educational development of hearing-impaired youngsters is thus essentially nonexistent.

There is also a concern for the amount of time the audiologist allots to informing key administrators about programs and services. Without taking time to work with these administrators, there is very little possibility for most educational audiologists to have a meaningful impact on the educational system in which they work; as with most systems, the status quo is the rule. Unfortunately, the current system is not adequately meeting the needs of hearing-impaired children.

Finally, it is abundantly clear that most educational audiologist feel little responsibility for the educational progress of hearing-impaired children in regular schools. The question must then be raised; Who has responsibility for the educational management of hearing-impaired children in regular schools? At the moment, that answer appears to be "no one." It is the contention of this book that the educational audiologist has the responsibility for managing the total spectrum of services for the hearing-impaired youngster. It may not be the responsibility of the audiologist to teach language, speech, reading, or other curricula, but it seems that the educational audiologist needs to coordinate services for the child in the mainstream so that there is unified effort to meet the hearing-impaired individual's educational and audiological needs. If there are no efforts made to improve the delivery of services, the authors believe that hearing-impaired youngsters in the regular schools will continue to fail to meet their potential.

REFERENCES

Allen W. Vision screening programs for hearing impaired children and youth. Paper presented at the International Convention of the Alexander Graham Bell Association for the Deaf, Houston, Texas, June, 1980, p.3.

American Speech-Language-Hearing Association. Ad Hoc Committee on Extension of Audiological Services in the Schools. ASHA, 1980, 22, 263–264.

Berg, F. Educational audiology: hearing and speech management. New York: Grune & Stratton, 1976.

Berg F & Blair J. Fault Tree analysis in educational audiology. Scientific exhibit, American Speech-Language-Hearing Association National Convention, Detroit, Michigan, Nov. 21–24, 1980.

Bess F & McConnell F. Audiology, education, and the hearing impaired child. St. Louis: C.V. Mosby Co., 1981.

Blair J. Effects of amplification, speechreading and classroom environments on reception of speech. Volta Review, 1977, 79, 443–449.

Blair J & Berg F. Problems and needs of hard-of-hearing students and a model for the delivery of services to the schools. ASHA, 1982, 24, 541–546.

Blair J, Peterson M, & Viehweg S. The effects of mild hearing loss on academic performance among young school-age children. Volta Review Feb 1985, 87, 87–94.

Blair J, Wright K, & Pollard G. Parental understanding of their children's hearing aids. Volta Review, 1981, 83, 375–382.

Clark T & Watkins S. The Ski*Hi model, programming for hearing impaired infants through intervention, home visits curriculum (4th ed.). Logan, Utah: Ski*Hi Institute, 1985.

Dalkey N. The Delphi method: An experimental study of group opinion (RM5888-PP). Santa Monica: Rand Corporation, June, 1969.

Davis J. Performance of young hearing impaired children on a test of basic concepts. Journal of Speech and Hearing Research, 1974, 17, 342–351.

Davis J, Shepard N, Stelmachowicz P & Gorga M. Characteristics of hearing impaired children in the public schools: Part II, psychoeducational data. Journal of Speech and Hearing Disorders, 1981, 46, 130–137.

Finitzo-Hieber T. Classroom acoustics. In R. Roeser & M. Downs (Eds.), Auditory disorders in school children. New York: Thieme-Stratton, 1981, pp. 250–262.

Finitzo-Hieber T & Tillman T. Room acoustics effects on monosyllabic word discrimination ability for normal and hearing impaired children. Journal of Speech and Hearing Research, 1978, 21, 440–458.

Gaeth J & Lounsbury E. Hearing aids and children in elementary schools. Journal of Speech and Hearing Disorders, 1966, 31, 283–289.

Jones K. The role of educational audiologists as viewed by school administrators, regular classroom teachers who serve hard-of-hearing children, and speech-language pathologists. Unpublished masters thesis, Utah State University, 1982.

Levine E. The psychology of deafness. New York: Columbia University Press, 1960.

Lillie D & Trohanis P. Teaching parents to teach. New York: Walker and Company, 1976.

Matkin N. Wearable amplification: A litany of persisting problems. In J Jerger (Ed.), Pediatric audiology, San Diego: College-Hill Press, 1984.

Matkin N, Hook P & Hixson P. A multidisciplinary approach to the evaluation of hearing-impaired children. Audiology, 1979, 4(7).

Mohindra I. Vision profile of deaf children. American Journal of Optometry and Physiological Optics, 1976, 53(8).

Myklebust H. The psychology of deafness. New York: Grune & Stratton, 1960.

Nault D. The effects of selected electroacoustic properties of FM systems on speech discrimination of moderately hearing impaired individuals in a reverberant classroom condition. Unpublished masters thesis, Utah State University, 1983.

Pollard G & Neumaier R. Vision characteristics of deaf students. American Annals of the Deaf, December 1974, pp. 740–745.

Quigley S & Thomure F. Some effects of hearing impairment upon school performance. In F N Martin (Ed.), Pediatric Audiology, Englewood Cliffs, N.J.: Prentice-Hall, 1978.

Roeser R & Downs M. Auditory disorders in school children. New York: Thieme-Stratton, 1981.

Roeser R & Nothern J. Screening for hearing loss and middle ear disorders in Rosser R & Downs M (Eds.). Auditory disorders in school children. New York: Thieme-Stratton, 1981.

Ross M with Brackett D, & Maxon A. Hard of hearing children in regular schools. New Jersey: Prentice-Hall, 1982.

Ross M. & Calvert D. Guidelines for audiology programs in educational settings for hearing impaired children. Volta Review, 79, 1977, pp. 153-161.

Ross M, & Giolas T. Auditory management of hearing impaired children. Baltimore: University Park Press, 1978.

Schlesinger H & Meadow K. Sound and sign. Los Angeles: University of California Press, 1972.

Shepard N, Davis J, Gorga M, & Stelmachowicz P. Characteristics of hearing impaired children in the public schools: Part I—Demographic data. Journal of Speech and Hearing Disorders, 1981, 46, 123–129.

Watkins S. Longitudinal study of the effects of home intervention on hearing impaired children. Unpublished doctoral dissertation, Utah State University, 1984.

Wilson-Vlotman A Practices and perceptions of educational audiology in the United States. Unpublished doctoral dissertation, Utah State University, 1984.

Witkin B & Stephens K. *Fault Tree analysis: A management science technique for educational planning and evaluation.* Technical Report No. 2, Hayward, CA: Alameda County School Department, 1973.

Yater V. Educational audiology. In J Katz (Ed.), *Handbook of clinical audiology,* (2nd ed.). Baltimore: Williams and Wilkins, 1978, pp. 589–595.

James C. Blair

3
Assessing the Hearing Impaired

As suggested in Chapter 2, it is important to assess the hearing impaired since many have problems in addition to that of hearing loss. Public Law 94-142 (Rules and Regulations of the Education of All Handicapped Children Act, 1975) stresses the importance of using a multidisciplinary team in the evaluation of handicapped children. The authors of this book also advocate the use of such a team, while realizing that this sort of team is not always used. The authors believe, however, that there is a need for someone in the schools who can overview the assessment process and who has the ability to synthesize assessment information in such a way that the data are interpreted correctly. It is the author's belief that the person who leads the team and/or collects the data needs to have a global view of hearing-impaired children and must understand the assessment process thoroughly. This book does not advocate that the assessment be done by the educational audiologist alone, but that this professional be in a position to screen problems that may be present and to seek help from other professionals in obtaining an accurate view of the youngster's current level of function. Shepard, Davis, Gorga, and Stelmachowicz (1981) point out in their report concerning the hearing impaired that too often there is limited or missing data in the files of hearing-impaired children. The findings of Shepard et al. highlight the need for a professional in the school system who is concerned about collecting accurate information so that appropriate programs may be planned. It is the author's view that the process of assessment ought to be similar to that proposed by Matkin, Hook and Hixson (1979). The assessment process consists of 3 parts: reports from parents and significant others; direct observations of the youngster being assessed; and the results from formal and informal tests. The authors also maintain that the use of a developmental model proposed initially by Myklebust (1954), and subsequently revised for this chapter is a simple, yet comprehensive, way to remember the scope of the assessment. There are 6 general areas of focus in the assessment model: perception, emotion, motor, intelligence, communication, and social adaptation. The first letters of these areas form the acronym "PEMICS", which is useful as a reminder of the global way to view youngsters in the evaluation process.

The PEMICS model will now be more fully explained. The area of perceptual testing (P) involves both auditory and visual assessment. As suggested by Allen (1980), there is a much higher incidence of visual problems among the hearing impaired than among the general population, and it is therefore important that children with hearing loss be screened visually to rule out visual problems. Of course, the auditory problems of the hearing impaired must also be given careful attention in order to help the hearing impaired compensate for their auditory impairments as much as possible.

The area of emotional (E) testing involves more than emotion alone; it includes the whole concept of psycho-social development. The literature suggests that hearing-impaired youngsters have significantly more psycho-social problems, particularly when mainstreamed into regular schools, than do normal hearing children (Myklebust, 1960; Schlesinger & Meadow, 1972; Sussman & Stewart, 1971). Blair (1983) asked teachers from 15 different school districts in Utah a question concerning the psycho-social adjustment of the hearing-impaired children with whom they worked in the regular schools. Seventy percent of the teachers (18 of 24 teachers) indicated that the hearing-impaired children with whom they worked had significant psycho-social problems.

The motor skills (M) of the hearing impaired are also more likely to be impaired than are the skills of normal hearing individuals. This is an area that needs considerably more research. Based on studies reported by Myklebust (1960), it can be said that the hearing impaired are less able to perform some motor tasks than are hearing people. For example, one area of primary concern was that of motor speed; the hearing impaired were not able to use their hands as quickly as were the normal hearing.

The intellectual (I) or cognitive abilities of the hearing impaired have been variously tested over a number of years (Moores; 1978; Quigley & Kretschmer, 1982; Quigley & Paul, 1984) and the basic findings suggest that there are differences in the function of hearing-impaired people on some tasks as compared to the function of the normal hearing, but that basically the hearing impaired are more like the hearing than they are different. It is clear, however, that the indiscriminate use of intelligence tests without an understanding of the role language plays in these measures will lead to faulty interpretation (Ross; 1982). Within the context of cognition, assessment is also made of learning abilities and of academic achievement.

Of course, the assessment of communication skills (C) of the hearing impaired is critical in the development of appropriate placement options as well as in the development of appropriate habilitative approaches. It is important to assess listening skills, speechreading abilities, and the ability to understand nonverbal cues, as well as the ability of these children to speak or communicate with others expressively in either verbal or nonverbal forms, including writing. Within the context of communication, reading abilities are also assessed.

Finally, it is critical that hearing-impaired youngsters be viewed in the context of their ability to successfully achieve independence, or social maturity (S). Too often there is a tendency to educate individuals in the context of the here and now and a failure to view the person in relationship to the world in which that person must learn to function. If youngsters are not able to compete successfully in their current placements, it is important to adjust the setting to the needs of these children, rather than the children to the needs of the setting. Some idea of how well these youngsters are doing in learning the basic skills of the society in which they live is also needed. The measurement of adaptive skills is thus an important part of the assessment process.

The process of assessment consists of 3 primary parts: obtaining information from the parents or significant others about youngsters being evaluated; observing children directly; and obtaining results from formal and informal tests.

PARENTS AND SIGNIFICANT OTHERS

Clark & Watkins, Introduction (1985) describe the importance of parents in the habilitation of hearing-impaired children. Watkins (1984) studied the long-term effects of parental intervention on the language learning of hearing-impaired children and found that parents are a significant variable in the success of such children over time. Parents also know more about their children and how they function than does anyone else. Yet, parents are often left out of the assessment process in favor of tests, which, as will be discussed later, are often faulty tools at best. If the goal is to obtain an accurate view of how children function, it is important to get information from parents or primary caregivers.

The first goal in meeting with the parents is to establish, as much as possible, an open, honest, collaborative relationship. The establishment of this relationship will make parents more likely to share perceived information and more able to accept the results of the assessment. Kübler-Ross (1969), Luterman (1979), and Moses (1979) all describe the grieving or mourning process in detail. The important issue for the educational audiologist to remember is that the grieving process is natural and that the only meaningful way to deal with this process is through acceptance of the parents' feelings. It is also important to remember, though, that unless parents are involved in the assessment process, it will frequently be impossible for them to accept the problem as reality. One of the important human principles to be kept in focus is that both parents, and professionals must be able to perceive a problem before that problem can be accepted as a reality. We have learned that until parents accept the problem as real or until the parent accepts the hearing loss or any other disability, the efficacy of any intervention program is minimal.

One of the ways the educational audiologist can foster collaboration is through learning what perceptions parents have about their children. It is important to both ask parents what concerns they have and to explain to them that the information they process about their child is very important to the assessment process (Cole & Wood, 1978). As the educational audiologist or multidisciplinary team proceeds through the assessment, one important objective is to verify the parents' perceptions as much as possible. This process assures that when the findings are presented, the results can be related to the parents in terms they understand; it can be pointed out that the information obtained verifies parental concerns. It is also important that the parents observe the assessment, if possible. This process again assures that, when findings are discussed, parents can relate these to the behaviors they observed during the assessment. The initial parent interview then provides the evaluator with a basic description of the youngster and the major symptomatology.

The Case History Interview

The case history interview is described in a number of places (Fuller, 1970; Myklebust, 1954; Rosenberg, 1978), and the authors do not intend to spend a great deal of time here on the details of the process. It is important, however, to keep the general outline of the case history in mind. Through the case history interview it is possible to obtain a view of the parents' current state of acceptance and a general overview of the youngster under study.

The interview typically begins with a question such as: "What concerns do you have about your child?" This question allows parents a chance to express their concerns and helps the assessor to understand what parents expect from the assessment. It is important for the assessor to answer parental questions as much as possible. Once parents' concerns have been established, additional information is obtained in order to establish a general overview of youngsters and how they relate to the PEMICS model described above. Typically, questioning would lead to obtaining specific information in the following areas: pregnancy and birth information; medical history; developmental history (auditory, motor, social and emotional, language and speech); educational experiences; cognitive development (use of senses, beginning use of symbols, logic, problem solving, reasoning); family history (names and ages of siblings, birth order of children, history of specific problems, socioeconomic status, educational background); social-psychological history (temperament and personality, playmates, difficulties, behavioral changes); auditory history (auditory responses to various stimuli, amplification that has been used, changes in auditory behavior over time); language and speech development; and current status (what youngsters are doing now).

It is likely that as a level of trust is reached between the parents and the interviewer, parents will feel free to ask questions. Parents are usually anxious to have their questions answered before the professional is really in a position to answer those questions accurately. Sometimes, however, the professional feels an obligation to answer parents' questions in order to reduce their anxiety. It is important to remember, however, that questions cannot be accurately answered until enough data have been collected. It is best to explain to the parents that the answers will be determined on the basis of the assessment, and that as answers are obtained they will be explained. It is also important to let parents know that any information they may remember about their child after the formal interview has finished should be shared with the assessor so that it can be taken into consideration in the assessment process. The goal of the assessor is to help parents realize that the assessment is a collaborative venture.

The educational audiologist needs to remember that in order for the interview to have a meaningful impact, the parent should do the talking and the educational audiologist the listening. As a general rule, parents can only hear what they are ready to hear. The parents will not remember much about the audiogram or much about the results of the assessment beyond the fact that their child is impaired and that there are some things that can be done to assist the youngster (Blair, Wright, & Pollard, 1981). It is also important to remember that parents have the responsibility for their children, and that, as a professional, the educational audiologist should inform, educate, and guide parents to appropriate sources of help and should support the parents as they grieve for the fact that their child has problems. Professionals need, however, to guard against assuming a parental responsibility.

Parent Education, Guidance, and Counseling

Matkin et al. (1979) propose some concepts which are useful as the role of educational audiologists with parents is addressed. As presented in the previous section, educational audiologists have a responsibility to help parents. The kind of help provided relates to 3 overlapping concepts: parent education, guidance, and counseling. As suggested earlier, in the initial assessment session it is important not to give the parents too much information; they cannot accommodate it. Probably the wisest course is to provide a limited amount of information concerning the findings that simply point out the major problems and to provide this briefly and without much embellishment. Before parents leave, they should be given information concerning how the educational audiologist can be reached and should be given the name of a parent of a child who has a similar problem. Another appointment to meet with the parents should be scheduled in about a week to 10 days. This initial stage is simply an informational and guidance stage. After parents have had some time to deal with the initial information and with the grieving process, they are then ready to receive additional information.

Again, it is important to wait for the parent to ask before a huge array of detailed information is presented. Generally speaking, by the second visit the parents are anxious to get more information. At that point, the audiologist can achieve a limited amount of education. It must be remembered, however, that questions must be answered in terms that the parents understand. If good a job was done in the case history interview, many of the parental perceptions will be known and the information provided to parents can be placed into a parental reference. For example, reference can be made to their observations as much as possible and the results of the assessment related to parental observation. i.e., "You indicated that Johnny responded to you by looking up when you walked into the room, but that he did not seem to hear the words you said. Our findings confirm your observations. Johnny is not able to hear conversational speech." This initial educational exchange should be followed with more formal educational meetings at a later time. It may be that the best way to educate parents is through groups or through parent home programs, such as that proposed by Clark and Watkins (1985). Part of the educational process involves teaching parents about hearing, hearing loss, and the effect of hearing loss on children and the family. Initial education should also cover intervention techniques, hearing aid management, and parental rights and responsibilities.

Parental guidance, as suggested above, may involve placing parents in contact with other parents who have had similar problems. Guidance will also entail directing parents to appropriate educational resources or other support agencies. Parents also need to be given sources of financial help and resources for additional testing, if appropriate. Often, parents who have their children in schools will become aware of Public Law 94-142 and may demand rights for their children, some of which may or may not be appropriate. The authors do have some concern at the moment regarding the inappropriate placement of the severely hearing impaired into regular classrooms. It is clear that the probability of these youngsters achieving maximum growth academically, socially, and emotionally in regular schools is very remote; yet, too often parents demand that their children be educated in the home school district, requiring that some makeshift services be provided and causing the children not to make the kind of adjustment the parents had intended. This is an issue that needs to be addressed by educators and parents so that handicapped individuals have a real chance to reach their maximum potential and to obtain a level of independence in their adult lives.

Parental counseling relates to the feelings of parents. Of course, audiologists are not trained to be counselors in the tradition of the psychotherapist.

Parents will, however, go to the person in the environment whom they can trust and can view as a significant individual. Audiologists who work in the schools are frequently viewed as significant others and therefore need to be prepared to deal with the issue of counseling. The kind of counseling that the educational audiologist will provide is that of support to parents. Active listening to the parents' expression of their feelings and helping parents sort out some of their feelings will be the kind of help the educational audiologist will provide. When parents get to the point where they do not seem to be making much progress and where they seem to have deeper problems than the educational audiologist can help, it is then necessary for the audiologist to seek out the help of a professional who can deal with these more serious issues. It seems, however that the audiologist working in the schools needs to be the kind of person who will take some time with parents and will listen to the parents' feelings and concerns. This will foster a reciprocal relationship that will ordinarily provide excellent dividends in terms of child growth.

OBSERVATIONS OF THE YOUNGSTER

Recall that in the assessment process there are 3 major parts: reports of parents and significant others (which have just been discussed); direct observation of the youngster being assessed; and formal and informal tests. This section will discuss observations of the youngster being assessed. Audiology is based on the scientific method and often it is perceived that the only accurate information is that which can be obtained through physical, objective measurement. Those who are the most skilled at assessment realize, however, that one of the primary tools available for accurate assessment is not in the test manual or in the test items, but are within the youngsters being assessed themselves. This type of assessment is not usually contained in the responses to test questions but in qualities and attributes presented by the individual. It is also true that the best diagnosticians have a very well developed feeling for children. They understand that the feelings they have about a youngster ought to be confirmed by test results, and parental observations. If test results contradict the feelings or the reports of parents or significant others, then the test results are questioned first. The results of tests are more likely to be wrong than are the careful observations of a good diagnostician.

Informal Observation

Observation of the youngster can be done under informal or formal conditions. Moses (1973) outlined the methods for this type of observation. He suggested that informal observation of the youngster take place in a relatively normal environment. For example, during recess there are many opportunities to observe the child informally. Another informal kind of observation can be accomplished under contrived conditions. For example, the youngster can be placed in a room with a fairly wide array of toys, such as trucks, playhouse, dolls and furniture, perhaps a sand table, playdough, building blocks, balls, and other toys that can be manipulated. These kinds of materials work well in the observation of youngsters from about 2 years of age to preadolescence. Older individuals might use paper, pencils (regular and colored), paint, puppets, or more sophisticated building materials (Erector sets, for example).

Youngsters are taken to a room where the examiner tells them to do anything they want for the next 30 minutes or so. The examiner observes youngsters in this setting without saying anything or doing anything with them unless something is requested. During this period, the examiner observes the following items

1. What types of activities seem to cause anxiety? The examiner needs to discover if this youngster is normally anxious about issues in the environment. Or do certain activities foster anxiety in the youngster? Or does it seem that nothing troubles this individual at all?

2. How does this individual solve problems? If this individual is observed in free interaction activities, there will be times of conflict over the choice of games or feelings about various issues. How does this individual look at these situations and solve them? Under contrived situations, when a child is presented with time to play in a relatively unfamiliar place, anxiety is common. The assessor can observe how the individual deals with this unnatural situation.

3. What independent learning skills are displayed? If the youngster begins to play a game or to engage intently in an activity, the individual will demonstrate some strategies that are used to interact with materials and activities available. By observing the youngster, it is possible to see what that child does and to observe whatever learning takes place. It is easy to observe whether the child is auditorily or visually oriented. It is also possible to observe whether the youngster spends a great deal of time with one thing or whether the child seems to wander from one activity to another without really spending any time in any one activity.

4. How quickly does the individual respond? The observation will reveal whether the youngster responds to things and/or to people. By placing an individual in a given environment with another person, ordinarily the person feels uncomfortable if nothing is said and will usually begin talking, even if the other individual is unknown. Children will behave in the same way; however, there is tremendous variability from individual to individual. Since the assessor is present in the room, the individual being tested is forced to deal with the assessor in some way, and watching this process provides information to the assessor on the quickness of response. Youngsters' interactions with other children in a play situation may also be observed.

5. How well does the individual attend to things? It is often a concern of

regular teachers that many of the hearing-impaired children with whom they work appear to have short attention spans. This may or may not be true. A number of hearing-impaired children really have excellent attention spans, but, because of their hearing loss, these youngsters scan the environment by using the visual sense. Those who hear normally also use a scanning procedure all the time, however, it is through the use of hearing. The normally hearing do not need to look around the environment to know what is going on—the ears do the scanning. When a youngster who is hearing impaired looks away from a speaker or a situation, it may simply be a normal response to the situation. On the other hand, it may be that the hearing-impaired child does have trouble attending to a situation for any length of time. Both unstructured and structured observations will allow the assessor to observe the youngster's attention span quite objectively.

6. Does the individual demonstrate abstract thinking? Observation of the child will often provide opportunities to observe the youngster engaging in various types of abstract thinking activities. Frequently, a youngster's play exhibits a high level of abstract thought during play with materials. For example, as subjects begin playing with objects, do they engage in play which is directly related to the object itself, or do they begin to create stories or fantasies that are only partly related to the object? Or perhaps there is no clear relationship between the object and the play, yet youngsters use the material in a highly creative way. The judgment of the subject's ability is often confirmed through more formal tests.

There are a variety of other qualities that can and will be observed during the informal observation period. The list above is only meant to provide tentative suggestions as to the range of possible observations that one might make. The important concept is that, through informal observations, a great deal can be learned about youngsters.

Structured Observation

The task in structured observation is to place the person being evaluated into a situation where the interaction is partially controlled. For example, a simple game is played with the subject, such as Old Maid or Go Fish. The goal in the games playing is to make certain that the youngster wins at least once and also loses at least once. The examiner is trying to observe what happens under both conditions. It is also important to learn how well the subject can engage in activities and interactions such as turn taking, cheating, authority delegation, and various kinds of structure.

Another situation that can be set up during the structured observation involves following directions. Can the subject listen to a relatively simple set of directions and follow them without difficulty? This information will aid tremendously in the formal testing situation. It will also provide more information on attention span, memory, and language.

One other task that might be set up in the structured observation time is the use of toys in prescribed ways. For example, Myklebust (1965) used a dollhouse with all the furniture and a sampling of family members in his structured play assessments. Under these conditions, youngsters are asked to organize the house in the way it should look. If subjects have trouble with the general instruction, more explicit instructions can be given, i.e.: "Here are some pieces of furniture that go into the kitchen; what rooms should have the other pieces of furniture?" It is also possible under this condition to have youngsters demonstrate some knowledge of interpersonal interactions in the home by the use of the family members. For example, it may be appropriate to ask subjects to show what mother does in the home and to then observe how youngsters manipulate the doll mother in the home setting. This information allows the examiner to see family interactions as they are perceived by subjects. It also allows the examiner to see the level of abstraction at which youngsters are functioning.

The results of the formal and informal observations should then be compiled by the examiner into some kind of gestalt and some general observations and conclusions should be drawn. The authors like the concept of Matkin et al. (1979) again, wherein they discuss the importance of a team meeting during the assessment process to assure that the information that has been obtained and questions that have been raised can be highlighted throughout the assessment. Recall that all the information obtained in the observations is as important as any other piece of information obtained throughout the assessment period. The formal tests, which will now be discussed ought, however, to confirm and amplify all other results obtained.

FORMAL AND INFORMAL TESTS

Purposes of Assessment

Before an appropriate test instrument can be selected, it is important to decide the purpose of the assessment. Salvia and Ysseldyke, p. 5 (1985), in their excellent book, suggest 5 purposes of assessment. The first purpose is screening. When screening, the examiner is interested in identifying those individuals who may be in need of more in-depth testing. When one selects a screening test, there is an automatic reduction in stringency in the test being employed. A screening test ought not be used as a diagnostic test; it is not designed for that purpose. The second purpose of assessment is placement. This type of assessment ought to be used to help educators select the placement which will most closely meet the total needs of the youngster. This type of testing ought not be designed, however, to justify a program into which the youngster could be placed. A third purpose of assessment is program planning, which is designed to help plan appropriate programs in subject areas such as reading, mathematics, etc. The assessment clarifies specific learning patterns that youngsters exhibit, so that appropriate educational intervention strategies may be planned. A fourth purpose of assessment is program evaluation; this is frequently used by school districts to determine if the children in the schools are learning as much as they should. The national study "A Nation at Risk" (1983) highlights this kind of assessment. The fifth purpose of assessment is to determine individual progress. The teacher is the person most often concerned with this area: "Are the children in my class learning anything?"

The purpose of the testing, to a large measure, determines the type of test that is best able to provide the information needed. The purpose also plays a large role in determining the level of validity and reliability that the examiner can accept in selecting a particular test. Since the educational audiologist will be in the position of interpreting test results, it is important that there be a basic understanding of the validity and reliability of the test instruments.

Selecting Tests

Validity

When designers of tests address the issue of validity, they are concerned with the concept of the test being able to measure what the authors or the users claim that the test measures. Validity is, however, a quality difficult to clearly prove. There are 3 types of validity: content validity, criterion-related validity, and predictive validity.

Content validity relates to 3 concepts: appropriateness, completeness, and level of mastery. The author and the individuals using the test are essentially left to decide this issue. For example, do the test items appear to be appropriate? Do the items seem to measure that which is relevant to the area being assessed? Do the test items really seem to measure the specific domain they are claimed to measure? It is amazing how often it is assumed that, because a test has a certain title, it in fact measures what it says it measures. For example, there are a variety of nonverbal tests available which in fact are not really nonverbal. The test items expect the person taking the test to be able to follow verbal directions. It is the examiner's responsibility to look at the test carefully before assuming it is, in fact, a valid test of what it purports to measure.

Another measure of a test's content validity is contained in the test's completeness. Again, the examiner is left to make this decision, although all test manuals should make some attempt to address this area in the test contents. It is important to understand what the limits of the test are, both in terms of the items selected and of the levels designed to be tested. The user must decide if the test really is broad enough to fully evaluate the subject's abilities, skills, and/or aptitudes.

Finally, a test's content validity should be evaluated in relation to the level of mastery being assessed. Bloom (1956), and Bloom, Hastings, and Madaus (1971) list 6 levels of mastery. The first level is knowledge. This level is focused on recall or recognition of specific elements in a subject area. Test questions at the level of knowledge will be very basic. A second level of mastery is comprehension. At this level, individuals are asked to reword information by putting a thought into their own words or by interpreting others ideas and seeing the interrelatedness between one set of ideas and another. A third level of mastery is application. The application level asks individuals to examine one set of ideas and to apply them to a different set. The fourth level of mastery is analysis, wherein an individual breaks down complex information into its component parts and, through this process, makes relationships between parts more clear. The fifth level is synthesis, wherein an individual examines parts, some of which may be very diverse, and puts them into a whole. Often, this latter process leads to the generation of a new idea that may not really be a sum of the whole, but, rather, an abstraction from the whole. The sixth and final level is that of evaluation. The task in evaluation is to make a judgment about the value of an idea, process, or product.

As can be seen from the above description, the concept of content validity is reasonably abstract and not always easy to determine without careful study of the test and the items that are contained in the test. Too often, tests are not carefully evaluated to determine if they are appropriate for use.

A second kind of validity is criterion-related validity. This can be broken into 2 components: concurrent validity and predictive validity. Concurrent validity relates to how well a person's test score can be used to estimate current levels of functioning. For example, how well does the score on the test agree with the teacher's perception of the student's present level of functioning? Or how well does the score on the test agree with other scores on similar tests, which are measuring the same thing? These data are usually reported in test manuals in terms of a correlation score, explaining that the scores on the present test agree with scores on a similar test at a certain level of reliability. Predictive validity is discussed in terms of how well the current score can predict performance at a later time. For example, the Graduate Record Examination (GRE) is used to predict how well a prospective student will do in graduate school. Intelligence tests are frequently used to predict how well individuals will do in school. Concurrent validity scores should be reported in the test manual.

A third type of validity is construct validity. Construct validity relates to the basic premises on which the test is based. For example, a construct for the Graduate Record Examination is that a person scoring at a level of 1000 or better will do well in graduate school. This construct is based on the theory that bright students with good verbal and quantitative skills score higher on the Graduate Record Examination than do students who are not bright. Research is then conducted on students in graduate programs to determine the relationship between scores on the GRE and grades, esteem of peers and professors, and clinical skills. All of this information should be reported about the test in order to examine the construct validity. Notice that the test sample does not include all people in the population and it may be that the construct on which the test is based is not true. Again, the user of the test must decide if the test is a valid test for the intended purposes.

Unfortunately, a number of tests currently being used may not have any of the types of validity cited above. It may be that, as Salvia and Ysseldyke (1985) suggest, the tests are being used on the basis of invalid types of data, i.e., cash validity, clinical utility, or internal consistency. Cash validity relates to the number of tests that have been sold or the number of tests being used in the field. Some of the producers of tests will claim the number of tests sold as a good criterion for the test's use; but, of course, in reality the number of tests sold has nothing to do with the validity of the instrument. Another kind of nonvalidity is clinical utility. When a publisher tries to sell a test on the basis of the usability of the test or its format, or on the basis of its appearance, then the focus is on clinical utility. It may be that a test is very easy to use and attractive to look at, but is totally invalid as a test instrument. Finally, the test may be considered valid on the basis of internal consistency. When addressing internal consistency, the focus is upon reliability, not validity. The responses to the items may be very repeatable and consistent throughout the test itself, but if the test does not measure what it purports to measure, it is not a valid test.

The concept of validity is important. The test administrator needs to be familiar with the test manual and must make a determination of the test's validity before using it in the assessment process. It also seems that educational audiologists should be in a position where they understand the tests that have been used and are able to give some suggestions concerning the appropriate tests to be used when assessing the hearing impaired. One of the purposes of this chapter is to help educational audiologists, or those working with the hearing impaired, to understand the process of assessment and to be able to interrelate with other professionals in making appropriate decisions about the educational management of the hearing impaired. Although the educational audiologist may not be trained to test all the areas described in the PEMICS model, the educational audiologist needs to understand what tests may be used and what they represent.

Reliability

A second major consideration in selecting or designing a test is that of reliability. When discussing reliability, one is interested in knowing that, if a tested trait is stable, a person will score the same on repeated testing. The more variation in an individual's scores from one occasion to another the lower the reliability. It is important for assessors to know when a *person* is variable versus the *scores on the test.* There are essentially 3 methods for determining reliability: test-retest reliability, alternate-form reliability, and internal consistency.

Test-retest reliability is based on a correlation between scores on the same test when 2 administrations are separated by a period of time. The level of correlation determines the degree of reliability. In contrast, alternate-form reliability is determined by developing 2 forms of the same test. One form of the test is administered to a large sample, and then the second form is administered to the same sample; the mean scores obtained from the 2 forms are then compared, along with the degree of variances between the 2 forms. The process is also repeated with another group with the same forms of the test being administered in the opposite order from that used for the first test group. Again, the mean scores and variances are compared between the forms. Finally, a process for determining internal consistency can be followed. Internal consistency may be the same as split-half reliability. For example, one can use a test that contains 20 items, if all the items measure the same trait or characteristic; 2 10-item tests can be developed from the same test. The 2 10-item tests are administered in the same way as that described for alternate-form reliability above, and the means and variances compared. Once the internal consistency is established, the test is considered reliable.

Salvia and Ysseldyke (1985) suggest 2 standards of reliability be used in determining if a test is reliable enough to warrant confidence in the results.

1. If the test scores are to be used for administrative purposes and are reported for groups, then a reliability correlation of about .60 should be the minimum level.

2. If a test score is to be used to make a decision about an individual student (e.g., placement in a particular class), then the level of reliability should be much higher, no lower than .90. On the other hand, if the purpose of the individual test is screening, the level of reliability may acceptably be .80 or greater.

In the judgment of the authors, it is too frequently assumed that a test used by the school, or by an assessor, is both reliable and valid. When the test manual is carefully examined, the test may be discovered to be neither. It is useful here to come back to a point made earlier: A test by itself is not the most reliable measure; in fact it is critical that the results of any one test not be accepted as the final word on a youngster's abilities. Any meaningful assessment should depend on a minimum of 2 tests that measure the same trait or ability, in addition to confirmation by parents and significant others as well as the direct observation of the youngster in both structured and unstructured situations.

Normative Data.

Another consideration in selecting a test is the normative data that were collected in order to develop the test. The reason for testing youngsters is to make certain kinds of inferences about individuals based on the results obtained. Final test items, however, are frequently selected on the basis of the statistics generated from the sample-population responses to original test items. For example, as a test is developed, a number of test items are included in the original test protocol and a target population is used to determine the difficulty of each item, i.e., which items are difficult for what age groups, or what items were missed by some subjects and not by others. Another reason that the normative sample is important is that an individual's performance on the test is evaluated in terms of the normative sample's performance. If the test norms are inadequate, the scores may be misleading. In order, therefore, for the test to be an accurate representation of an individual's abilities, the normative population used for the development of the test must be representative. The adequacy of a test's norms depends on 3 factors: representativeness of the normative sample, the number of cases in the normative sample, and the relevance of the norms in terms of the purpose of the test.

The representativeness of a population is based on 2 considerations:

1. Does the normative sample contain some of the same kinds of people as the population that the norms are intended to represent? Are subjects present with the same level of maturation, same skills, race, intelligence, etc. as are in the general population?

2. Are various kinds of people present in the same proportion in the sample as they are in the population of reference? The normative sample must have the correct proportions of ethnic and racial groups, as well as appropriate numbers of males and females, and correct representation of the geographical areas of the people represented in the sample.

Another consideration in the normative sample is the number of subjects in the sample. In order for a sample to be representative at all there must be at least 100 individuals for each of the levels included in the test. For example, if the test is based on age norms, there must be 100 subjects for each of the ages represented in the test. This sample must then be distributed in accordance with the considerations suggested above.

Finally, it is important to examine the norms in terms of their relevance to the purpose of the testing. Even if the test is normed appropriately for the sample in the test, it still may not be truly representative of the subjects in the locality in which the youngster being evaluated will be expected to function. For example, Blair, Peterson, and Viehweg (1985) examined the scores of mildly impaired youngsters on a national scale versus the youngsters' scores when compared to their hearing peers in regular classrooms; they found significant differences between the 2 comparisons. If the assessor is interested in determining how a given student will function in a local school, it is best to compare the youngster with peers in the local school rather than with the national population.

For a more thorough treatment of the issues described in this section,

Salvia and Ysseldyke's (1985) book should be read. Attention will now be shifted to the assessment of each of the areas addressed in the PEMICS model described earlier.

PERCEPTUAL TESTING

The first general area for assessment in the PEMICS model is perception. The area of perception is divided into 2 subsections: vision and audition. Visual screening will be discussed first and then auditory perceptual screening will be examined.

Visual Screening

Myklebust (1960) reported that hearing-impaired individuals have a higher incidence of visual perception problems, more color blindness, and more visual defects than do the normal hearing. Alexander (1973), Mohindra (1976), Pollard and Neumaier (1974), and Suchman (1967) all suggest that children with hearing loss have more problems visually than does the normal hearing population. Unfortunately, there are a limited number of test protocols being used in the United States that routinely recommend that a thorough vision screening test be done on hearing-impaired children. This appears to be a fairly serious oversight on the part of educators and evaluators. Youngsters with hearing impairment are very dependent on visual abilities to help enhance their receptive language capabilities as well as to enable reading and a great many educational tasks. Allen (1980) suggested a screening program that the authors believe has merit and should be used more widely for vision screening in hearing-impaired youngsters.

The most typical visual screening test is the Snellin chart at 20 feet. The visual test that most people pass, however, is the far-seeing acuity test (Salvia and Ysseldyke, 1985). On the other hand, the kind of testing done less often is of near visual abilities—yet the skills that youngsters need the most in order to do well in school are near visual skills. It seems that the place where screening for visual problems could most logically occur is in the schools. As explained earlier, Allen (1980), suggests that visual screening be done on a routine basis.

One kind of screening recommended is eye movement skill (ocular motility) screening. This screening focuses on the ability to move the eyes quickly and to control visual inspection. The task here is to watch youngsters while they are reading and observe whether eye movements are slow, clumsy, or uncoordinated. For example, if the eyes jump, miss, or seem to stutter, or if youngsters seem to lose their place while reading, then there will, in all likelihood, be a reduction in reading speed and comprehension. If the teacher, educational audiologist, or other professional observes these problems, it would be wise to refer the children for a more complete eye examination.

There are a number of symptoms present when youngsters have ocular motility problems. One symptom is that visually demanding materials are avoided. It is not uncommon for these youngsters to be labeled as behavior problems, because in order to avoid reading materials, they use secondary behaviors to help delay the punishment encountered in reading. These youngsters may thus act out or exhibit avoidance behaviors. For example, youngsters with visual problems may indicate a need to sharpen a pencil several times whenever a visual motor task is expected, or youngsters may need to go to the bathroom, or may cause problems by talking with other children, or perhaps cause disruptions of various kinds. These children are often labeled as troublemakers; the real problem is not identified. Another symptom frequently exhibited is an increase in head turning while reading. These youngsters may demonstrate shorter attention spans for visual materials than for other kinds of activities. Finally, these students may show an increase in fatigue and restlessness during all types of continued visual activities.

A second problem is eye teaming skills (binocularity). For most of us, both eyes perform as one; however, there are a number of youngsters who do not have eye teaming abilities. When there is no binocularity, there are problems with spatial orientation, depth perception, seeing clear relationships between symbols, and seeing symbols clearly. This problem leads to difficulty in perceiving near-point, visually demanding materials. Youngsters without good binocularity will show preference for and skill in listening activities, but will avoid visual activities. Professionals are encouraged to watch children read to be sure both eyes are being used together.

A third type of visual problem is that of eye-hand coordination. Much of what is expected of youngsters in school is dependent on the use, practice, and integration of the eyes and hands as paired learning tools. Through this skill emerges the ability to make visual discriminations regarding size, shape, texture, and location of objects, as well as the ability to produce drawn and written symbols. Youngsters who have problems with eye-hand coordination demonstrate extreme lack of orientation to the page, have difficulty staying within the lines when writing, or perhaps demonstrate an inability to use their hands to help control the movement of the writing instrument. Use of the Beery Buktenica Test of Visual Motor Integration (Beery & Buktenica, 1967) is recommended for this problem, as well as observation of the youngster in school-related activities that demand eye-hand coordination.

A fourth type of problem is visual form perception (visual comparison, visual imagery, and visualization). Visual form perception is a derived skill, not a separate and independent ability. The purpose of visual form perception is to discriminate, quickly and accurately, visual likenesses and differences. The usual symptoms seen with youngsters who experience poor visual form perception are confusion in seeing similarities, inattention to slight differences that make a significant difference (word choice, for example), reversals of letter forms, and/or use of letter sequences that are not phonetically related. Youngsters with visual-form perception problems are often judged to have a poor memory or to be careless about details. Zieziula' (1982) recommends the Motor-Free Visual Perception Test (Colarusso & Hammill, 1972) as a way to screen for visual perception. There appears to be fairly wide use of the Detroit Test of Learning Aptitude (Barker & Bernice, 1967), at least the use of some of the subtests related to visual perception and wide use of some subtests from the Woodcock-Johnson Psychoeducational Battery (Wood-cock, 1978).

A fifth area of concern is refraction status (nearsightedness, farsighted-ness, focus problems). The test most often used to identify youngsters with these kinds of problems is the Snellin Wall Chart, which, as suggested above probably finds the problem which least affects activities most frequently encountered in school. Tools which would identify more problems are the Keystone Telebinocular and the Bausch and Lomb Orthorater (Salvia & Yss-eldyke, 1985).

Finally, an area that needs to be evaluated is colorblindness. The use of color in the development of textbooks and various kinds of teaching materials is widespread in education today. Usually, the use of these materials will not be a serious problem, but there are some youngsters who find it difficult to see some materials using colors which are not visible to the colorblind indi-vidual. In screening for colorblindness, Salvia and Ysseldyke (1985) recom-mend the use of at least 2 tests. The most commonly used tests are the Farnsworth Dichotomous Test for Color Blindness (Farnsworth, 1947), the AO H-R-R Pseudoisochromatic Plates (Hardy, Rand, & Rittler, 1957), and the Ishihara Color Blindness Test (Ishihara, 1970).

Auditory Screening

A complete discussion of auditory screening is presented in Chapter 4. This section will briefly explore the area of auditory perceptual or central auditory difficulties. The authors suggest 2 references be examined in order to obtain a greater understanding of auditory perceptual difficulties: Keith (1977, 1981) or Northern and Downs (1984). It is important to realize, however, that the study of auditory perceptual difficulties is of recent origin, and, as with any new area of study, there is a period of research and development that occurs before the most appropriate diagnostic and habilitative ap-proaches are clearly identified. In the meantine, professionals working with youngsters in the schools are in a position where they must try to identify the youngsters who have problems and to do everything in their power to help them make maximum adjustment to the world in which they live.

The area of greatest controversy in auditory perceptual problems relates to the basic question of cause: Do auditory perceptual problems cause language difficulties or do language difficulties or deficits cause auditory perceptual problems? The problems of auditory deficits which were described by Myklebust (1954) are very much in evidence, but the treatment of these problems is not well substantiated at this time. It has been found that some children with whom the authors work have made significant growth when treatment of the auditory problems appears to be appropriate to the youngster. It has also been found, however, that a number of children appear to make little or no change after treatment. It is hoped that considerable progress will be made during the next few years and that a wider array of materials will be available from which to choose in assisting children who exhibit these problems.

It is the author's belief that children who have symptoms suggesting auditory perceptual difficulties should be helped as much as possible by professionals in the field. In order to provide assistance, these children must be identified. A number of tools have been developed to assess youngsters who have auditory perceptual difficulties. One method of assessment involves the use of a checklist for a teacher to screen children class. A checklist might include items suggested by Cohen (1980), e.g.:

1.   The children have normal pure-tone hearing.
2.   They respond inconsistently to auditory stimuli.
3.   They have short attention spans and tire easily when confronted with long or complex activities.
4.   They are easily distracted by both auditory and visual stimuli.
5.   They frequently have difficulty localizing sounds in the environment, including the ability to detect how near or far the sound source is located, or the differences between soft and loud sounds.
6.   They may listen closely, but have difficulty following long or complicated verbal commands or instructions.
7.   They often request that information be repeated.
8.   They are often unable to remember information presented verbally, both long-term and short-term.
9.   They are often allergic to various things in the environment.
10. They often have a significant history of chronic otitis media.

The authors' experience suggests that the use of parents and teachers in the process of evaluation of central auditory problems raises the problem of getting the cooperation of these significant individuals in the intervention program. With the cooperation of parents and teachers, long-term growth effectiveness is significantly enhanced for the hearing impaired youngster. In addition to the checklist procedure described above, Keith (1977, 1981) describes most common areas that test developers try to measure. These include:

Auditory Attention. This is the ability to sustain attention over a period of time. The youngster ought to be able to direct attention to an acoustic stimulus for a time that is similar to that exhibited by other youngsters of the same age.

Auditory Figure Ground. This is the ability to understand or repeat an auditory stimulus presented in a background of competition (speech or noise). An individual will ordinarily be able to understand a speech signal in a background of noise quite easily, provided the noise is a little less intense than the background. Youngsters with central auditory problems have considerable difficulty even in a relatively quiet setting. In other words, even a little background noise affects their ability to discriminate speech.

Auditory Discrimination. This is the ability to hear whether spoken speech sounds are the same or different or to identify words that are phonemically similar through either speech repetition or picture pointing.

Auditory Closure. This is the ability to understand the whole word or message when part is missing or missed.

Auditory Blending. This is the ability to hear the parts of words and to synthesize them into a whole. It is postulated by Bannatyne (1971) that auditory blending and closure abilities are closely related.

Auditory Analysis. This is the ability to identify phonemes, syllables, or morphemes embedded in words.

Auditory Memory. This is the ability to hold words, ideas, or other auditory stimuli for a period of time and then repeat them back in sequence or perhaps numerical order.

Sequential Memory. This is the ability to hold sequences of auditory stimuli in an exact order. The stimuli usually used to assess sequential memory are digits (Keith, 1981).

The reader should observe that many of the skills listed above are overlapping and that the separation of these tasks into unique entities is not possible. Audiometric tests are also used to measure auditory processing abilities; the reader is referred to Keith (1977, 1980, 1981) for a complete description of these procedures.

It is the authors' recommendation that if central auditory difficulties are suspected, the youngster should be evaluated by an audiologist who specializes in central auditory assessment and also by a learning disability specialist who can perform the kinds of educational tests suggested above.

EMOTIONAL ASSESSMENT

The second area to be assessed following the PEMICS model is emotion. The kind of assessment that focuses on emotion is usually described as a personality assessment.

Personality Tests

Each of us develops a view of the world based on a variety of experiences. As we interact with other people, we develop a basic sense of who we are, what our abilities are, and how we present ourselves to the world. Most of us develop a consistent pattern of response to others and become, to a large degree, predictable. This presentation to the world gradually evolves into a way of behaving that is usually referred to as our personality. Because personality is based on behavior, it is possible to describe personality in terms of typical or normal behaviors. Battin (1981) suggests that personality tests are designed to provide information about the individual's perception of the world, how that individual copes, the individual's social skills, self concept, and frustration tolerance level. There are basically two different kinds of psychological tests: objective and subjective. The objective test usually asks subjects to give yes/no responses or some other response which is easily scored (true/false or multiple choice). Subjective tests are based on personal interpretation and response. These kinds of tests are not as easy to score. Personality tests of a subjective nature are tests such as Thematic Apperception Test (Murray, 1943), the Hand Test (Bricklin, Zygmunt, & Wagner, 1981), the House-Tree-Person Test (Buck & Jolles, 1966), and the Rorschach Test (Rorschach, 1966).

The research literature on the personality characteristics of the hearing impaired has been seriously flawed by the use of personality tests which require substantial verbalizations in order to be interpreted; therefore, the results have been questionable. Additionally, many of the studies have been done with the perceptions of others about the hearing impaired, a practice which may not be truly indicative of any emotional problems per se, but, rather, of a non-handicapped person's ability to accept a handicapped person. In addition to these concerns, there is a considerable criticism of projective tests and most personality tests because of problems in validity and reliability. Despite these limitations, the literature reports essentially the same results using different tests (Levine & Wagner, 1974; Schlesinger & Meadow, 1972).

Levine (1976) summarizes the general emotional patterns of the hearing impaired as being emotional immaturity, adaptive rigidity, sociocultural impoverishment, and narrowed intellectual functioning. Kretschmer and Quigley (1981) add short attention span and poor impulse control as 2 additional personality traits. In reality, as Levine (1976) suggests, it is inappropriate to expect that there be one typical personality of the deaf, because the hearing-impaired population is a very heterogeneous group. As Levine studied different youngsters who functioned in different ways, she discovered significant differences between groups of hearing-impaired children. Maxon, Brackett, and van den Berg (1982) also have discovered that mainstreamed hearing-impaired children are really more like normal hearing individuals than they are different. In all probability, the differences discovered are due more to healthy adjustment to a handicap than to any significant emotional problem. It is still true, however, that a number of hearing-impaired individuals are likely to suffer the same kinds of emotional problems as are present in the hearing population. Rainer and Altshuler (1967) report that there are no more seriously mentally ill individuals in the hearing-impaired population than there are in the normal hearing population; the likelihood of discovering the serious problems among the hearing impaired is just as possible as among the normal hearing.

McCrone (1979) reported that a number of hearing-impaired youngsters develop what he identified as "learned helplessness". Learned helplessness is defined by 3 characteristics: an external locus of control; underachievement; and reduced performance when faced with failure. Impulsive behavior and the ability to take responsiblity for individual action are both qualities that can be modified by a person. Since the hearing impaired have difficulty with these areas, it is appropriate to assess impulsivity and responsiblity.

The evaluation of emotional health, then, is one of the areas that needs to be examined. There are, however, some problems in assessing this area with a high degree of reliability and the area of emotion is often avoided because it is too nebulous or because evaluators are afraid that they may in fact discover a problem and not know what to do. In spite of the difficulties of assessment, if a youngster is discovered to have a significant emotional problem, it is possible to provide some help for this youngster through appropriate intervention. The intervention can psychologically help individuals develop a more productive and enjoyable life than might be true without intervention. It will be a mistake to fail to provide help to youngsters who need it.

The authors suggest that hearing-impaired youngsters be screened for significant problems in the area of emotional health. As described earlier, one of the important ways to assess individuals for problems is through direct observation of these youngsters in both formal and informal settings. Through careful observation, emotional problems are often discernable. It is important when a problem is suspected that the school psychologist or other mental health professional be invited to evaluate the youngster in-depth.

Assessment Battery

It is the authors' view that the most appropriate way to discover emotional problems is to observe youngsters as they relate with other students in the environment and as they relate with teachers and parents. It is also appropriate to observe youngsters in both structured and unstructured situations. There are, however, a number of tests that can be administered to confirm the impressions generated by such observations. The House-Tree-Person Test (Buck & Jolles, 1966) has been successfully used with the hearing impaired, as has the Hand Test (Wagner, 1983), the Draw-A-Person Test (Urban, 1963), and the Rotter Incomplete Sentences (Rotter, 1966). In assessing impulsivity and locus of control, Kretschmer and Quigley (1981) suggest the following 6 tests: Matching Familiar Figures Test (Chandler, 1975); Timed Draw-A-Man Test; Porteus Mazes; Wechsler Mazes; Id-Ego-Superego Test; and the Rotter Test of Internal/External Control.

Waller, Sollad, Sander, and Kunicki (1983) suggest that emotional problems might also be identified through the use of checklists and personality questionnaires. Waller et al. suggest the Louisville Behavior Checklist (Miller, 1977) and the Burks Behavior Rating Scale (Burks, 1977) as good tools to be used in the schools. They also recommend the use of the Early School Personality Questionnaire (Coan & Cattell, 1976).

MOTOR FUNCTIONING

The third area to be assessed in the PEMICS model is motor functioning.

When individuals have processing deficits in one modality there is an increased probability that these individuals will demonstrate impairments in another modality (Wyatt, 1969). For example, youngsters with auditory disorders often demonstrate a higher-than-normal incidence of problems in motor skills and visual motor skills (Myklebust, 1960). Unfortunately, there has not been very much research done on the hearing-impaired in the motor area; extensive research needs to be completed. Ayres (1972) has worked in the motor area with normal and learning-disabled youngsters and an increasing number of occupational therapists are being employed by schools of the deaf and in special programs for the handicapped. This is a good sign for the special programs; unfortunately, youngsters in the regular schools do not usually receive the services of professionals trained to work with motor problems.

Hearing loss may affect motor development from at least 2 viewpoints. First, hearing loss by its very nature affects the integrity of the central nervous system and the semicircular canals. The effects in the motor area of the central nervous system will, in many instances, affect the gross motor abilities of the hearing impaired, i.e., balance, locomotion, and speed of motor movement. Myklebust (1960) reported that the deaf performed the same as the hearing in sitting, walking, dexterity, and synkinesia (involuntary movement). The deaf, however, functioned at a level significantly below that of the hearing in the development of laterality, simultaneous movement, locomotor coordination, balance, and speed of motor movement.

A second way in which a profound hearing loss may affect motor abilities is through the lack of hearing itself. It may be that, because hearing-impaired individuals cannot hear certain features in the environment, they perform some motor tasks in a way different than that of the normal hearing. For example, deaf individuals often shuffle their feet as they walk. Instead of lifting their feet above the ground in firm steps, the deaf tend to skim the surface of the ground, walking with a shuffle. It has been postulated by Myklebust (1960) that the shuffling gait is a result of not hearing the sound of the footsteps, or perhaps a result of the need for more tactile information in order to maintain appropriate balance because of central nervous system dysfunction.

Assessing Motor Abilities

As suggested above, testing for motor problems has not been well developed or researched. Billiar (1983) describes some of the signs of gross and fine motor difficulties, as well as some of the signs of visual motor problems. It is important that professionals working with hearing-impaired individuals be alert to the possibility of problems in motor abilities and therefore understand some motor problem symptoms.

Signs of Gross Motor Difficulties. Individuals with motor problems will exhibit a developmental delay motorically, i.e., a delay in sitting, walking, running, and other types of motor tasks. As youngsters grow older, there may be a number of signs of motor difficulty. For example, if youngsters are more clumsy than normal, or if they drop things, trip a lot, or perhaps fall more frequently than do other children, there are perhaps motor problems present. It is also possible that these youngsters have problems with spasticity or decreased muscle tone. A number will also have problems in motor planning, i.e., controlling the direction and position of arms, hands, or fingers in space. They may also have general muscle weakness, slow, labored motor movements, poor posture, difficulties isolating motor movements, and, finally, overflow from one side of the body to the other. All these problems might be reduced with the help of trained professionals in the motor area.

Signs of Fine Motor Difficulties. The symptoms of fine motor problems are poor grasp of a pencil (ages 4–5 or older), inability to point to a picture (ages 1½ and older), perseveration of motor movements, difficulty planning fine motor movements, weakness in the hands, and slow, labored movement of the hands. Again, these difficulties might be reduced with appropriate intervention.

Signs of Visual/Perceptual Difficulties. The symptoms of visual/perceptual difficulties include the inability to pick out the parts of a picture (ages 3–4 and older), the inability to copy or print from a model, holding a paper too close or too far away, reaching out for a step before going down, and missing or falling off a step or a chair.

Formal Tests. Probably the best general test of motor proficiency is the Bruininks-Oseretsky Test of Motor Proficiency (1978). This test is designed to yield 3 estimates of motor proficiency: a gross motor composite score; a fine motor composite score; and a total composite score. The gross motor section consists of 4 subtests which provide an index of the ability to use the large muscles effectively. The fine motor composite consists of 3 subtests which provide an index of the ability to use the small muscles of the lower arm and hand effectively. The gross and fine motor skills are measured in one subtest. The battery composite section summarizes performance on all 7 subtests which provide an index of general motor proficiency. There are both short and long form versions of the test. The test is designed for use with youngsters between the ages of 5 and 15 years.

A number of school districts and educational programs have developed their own motor tests, which appear to be viable as a means of screening for problems in the area of motor proficiency. For example, Smith (1967) developed a Perceptual Motor Test to screen for problems in the areas posture, balance, coordination, awareness, and patterned movements. The Denver Developmental Screening Test (Frankenburg & Dodds, 1970) has also been used to evaluate, at least in a general way, both fine and gross motor skills. A test that has been used to evaluate visual amotor development is the Developmental Test of Visual-Motor Integration (Beery & Buktenica, 1967). This test is designed for use with youngsters between the ages of 2 and 15.

The authors recommend that youngsters with hearing loss be carefully evaluated in the area of motor proficiency to determine if there are problems. As suggested earlier, recognition of deficient functioning and appropriate assessment of all aspects of the person should be a part of the differential diagnostic process.

INTELLIGENCE TESTING (COGNITION)

The fourth area to be assessed in the PEMICS model is the area of intelligence or cognition. The formal assessment of this area needs to be carried out by a trained professional, usually a psychologist, psychiatrist, or psychometrist. It is, however, important that professionals working with the hearing impaired understand how this testing is done, what tests should be used, and what the results mean, in order that appropriate educational decisions be made.

Intelligence

The measurement of intelligence originated recently with the development of intelligence tests in 1900. It is probably not possible, however, to accurately measure all the aspects of intelligence, since the sum of the parts is not equal to the whole. Additionally, intelligence may in reality be directly related to the sociocultural environment rather than to test-taking abilities.

For example, an individual living in a low socioeconomic environment may need to learn some cognitive problem-solving strategies that are totally unknown to an individual living in a higher socioeconomic environment, and vice versa. The abilities of these 2 individuals will probably be significantly different in regard to test-taking abilities, as well as different in their abilities to do well in their respective environmental circumstances. As viewed on the basis of criterion validity, i.e., success in school versus scores on a test, intelligence tests do, on the average, provide some predictive information (better in predicting reading grades than predicting geometry grades). Salvia and Ysseldyke (1985) point out that even in the area of criterion validity, however, intelligence tests are not even close to accurately predicting success in school as much as 70 percent of the time. In other words, if a youngster obtains a high intelligence test score, there is still a very good chance that the youngster may not do well academically.

Intelligence testing with the hearing impaired has created controversy, beginning in 1930 with the suggestion by Patterson and Williams that the hearing impaired had lower intellectual ability than did normal hearing individuals. Vernon (1969) reported that the results of approximately 50 independently conducted investigations showed that the hearing impaired are essentially the same as the hearing, intellectually. The language deficits of the hearing impaired interfere, however, with their ability to do well on verbal tests of intelligence. It is probably wise to view intelligence testing as a test of an individual's strengths and weaknesses in certain areas as measured by the test, and not to be too concerned about intellectual function, unless there is information about the individual that suggests that, in addition to the hearing loss, there truly is a cognitive deficiency. The decision that a youngster is intellectually inferior should only be made when at least 2 measures of nonverbal intelligence suggest a significant deficit and when the youngster's demonstrated abilities as reported by the teachers and the parents confirm that the youngster is low in the cognitive domain.

For the average hearing-impaired youngster who will be successfully placed in the regular school, the authors are most concerned about 2 questions: How well can this youngster compete with hearing youngsters in a regular school setting? What are this youngster's strengths and weaknesses? In order to clearly answer these 2 questions, it is the authors' view that tests should be used that sample a wide array of abilities. Although the Leiter International Performance Scale (Leiter, 1949; Arthur, 1950), the Goodenough-Harris Drawing Test (Goodenough & Harris, 1963), the Ravens Progressive Matrices (Raven, Court, & Raven, 1977), and the Chicago Nonverbal Examination (Brown, Stein, & Rohrer, 1947) have all been used to assess the intelligence of the hearing impaired by a variety of researchers, the authors believe that these measures, although reliable, are not necessarily the most valid tools available to sample the learning skills or learning aptitudes of the hearing impaired if the goal of the assessment is to obtain information to aid in placement decisions or in educational strategies. The authors' experience suggests that the Wechsler Scales (Adult Intelligence Scale [WAIS], 1981; Intelligence Scale for Children [WISC-R], 1974; Preschool and Primary Scale of Intelligence [WIPPSI], 1967) are good tools to use, particularly for mainstreamed hearing-impaired students, and that the Hiskey-Nebraska Test of Learning Aptitude (Hiskey, 1966) is a good test to use.

Recall, the preferred tests are preferred not because they measure cognition or intelligence most fairly, but, rather, because the tests allow assessors to discover strategies that youngsters use in performing a variety of diverse cognitive tasks. For example, the Wechsler scales are comprised of 2 sections: a performance section and a verbal section. Each section is further divided into subtests. The verbal sections of the Wechsler tests consist of subtests such as:

Information. This subtest assesses the ability to answer specific factual questions.

Comprehension. This subtest assesses the ability to comprehend verbal directions or to understand specific customs and mores.

Arithmetic. This subtest assesses the ability to solve problems requiring the application of arithmetic operations.

Vocabulary. This subtest assesses the ability to define words verbally.

Similarities. This subtest assesses the ability to identify similarities or commonalities in superficially unrelated verbal stimuli.

The performance section of the Wechsler tests consists of subtests such as:

Picture Completion. This assesses the ability to identify missing parts in pictures.

Picture Arrangement. This assesses comprehension, sequencing, and identification of relationships by requiring the subject to place pictures in sequence to produce a logically correct story.

Block Design. This assesses the ability to manipulate blocks in order to reproduce a visually presented stimulus design.

Object Assembly. This assesses the ability to place disjointed puzzle pieces together to form a complete object.

Coding, or Digit Symbol, or Animal House. These are different subtests on the various Wechsler tests that measure the ability to associate certain symbols with others and to copy them on paper.

Both sections of the test are used together to obtain a view of an individual's global intelligence. Obviously, the hearing-impaired youngster may be expected to do significantly better on the performance section than on the verbal section. If one is not concerned with intelligence per se, however, but with a particular youngster's ability to solve problems when compared with hearing youngsters, the Wechsler tests can serve as an excellent tool.

Another test the authors use, and find to be a valuable asset, is the Hiskey-Nebraska Test of Learning Aptitude (Hiskey, 1966). This test has been standardized for both the hearing and the deaf. It is possible to give either pantomime or verbal directions when administering the test. It is not necessarily the best measure of intelligence, since there are a number of technical errors in the data reported for the test. But in the authors' experience, it is an excellent tool for assessing learning strategies for youngsters between the ages of 5 and 12 years. The reason this test is preferred is that it evaluates the subject over 12 different subtests. The kinds of tasks required of each subject are:

Bead Patterns. This assesses short-term visual memory, motor speed, and visual perception.

Memory for Color. This assesses visual memory and sequencing skills.

Picture Identification. This assesses matching skills and visual perception.

Picture Association. This assesses the ability to perceive conceptual relationships between pictorial ideas. In order to complete this task, a youngster must be able to make generalizations.

Paper Folding. This assesses matching abilities and visual, spatial memory.

Visual Attention Span. This assesses sequencing abilities and memory.

Block Patterns. This assesses spatial ability, motor speed, and how an abstract shape is related to a concrete object.

Completion of Drawings. This assesses visual perception, awareness of the environment and visual motor abilities.

There are additional items for older subjects, but the foregoing provides the reader with a general idea of the breadth of the test.

As suggested earlier, the primary task of the assessor is to identify the areas that will help youngsters achieve well in school and also to identify, as clearly as possible, what areas will potentially cause problems as youngsters try to compete with normal hearing students in the regular classroom. The selection of those tests that measure the greatest number of skills seems to be the most useful.

COMMUNICATION ASSESSMENT

The fifth area in the PEMICS model is that of communication. The assessment of the communicative skills of the hearing impaired have been addressed by a number of researchers (Brackett, 1982; Kretschmer & Kretschmer, 1978; Moeller, 1984; Moeller, McConkey, & Osberger, 1983, 1981; Ross, 1982; and a number of others). It is not the purpose of this section to fully explore the topic of communication assessment, but only to provide an overview of the process that has been found to be helpful in the evaluation of communication skills. The schema the authors like is that described by Brackett (1982). Brackett divided the communication assessment into 6 areas: the reception of spoken language; the comprehension of spoken language; the production of spoken language; the production of speech; the comprehension and production of written language; and communicative competence. Each of these areas will be discussed separately.

The Reception of Spoken Language

Look/Listen/Look and Listen.   One of the pieces of information that educators need to know is what modality or modalities a particular youngster uses in receiving spoken information. As suggested in Chapter 5, sometimes audiologists are so concerned about the pure-tone, impedance, speech, and other results, that they fail to obtain the information that can help the teacher in providing the best possible educational input to the youngster. The assessor needs to gather information on how well the youngster receives information when it is presented auditorially alone, versus when it is presented visually alone, versus when it is presented in an auditory visual mode. The assessor must also learn how well the subject can receive this information in a background of noise. The intent of this kind of testing is to help the educator understand how information can be presented to the youngster in the most effective manner. Chapter 6 details the assessment of listening skills in detail.

In order to test ability to receive spoken language, a number of materials have been developed. There are word lists that are equivalent and appropriate to use with children with varying amounts of receptive language abilities, i.e., PBK lists (Haskins, 1949), NU CHIPS lists (Elliott & Katz, 1980), WIPI lists (Ross & Lerman, 1971), and CID lists (Hirsh, Davis, Silverman, Reynolds, Eldert, & Benson, 1952), which are probably the most widely used. If the assessor is interested in using sentences, there are a few sentence lists that have been developed and used in assessing the ability to receive spoken language: WIPI sentences (Weber & Reddell, 1976), SPIN sentences (Kalikow & Stevens, 1977), CID everyday sentences (Silverman & Hirsh, 1955), Blair sentences (Blair, 1976), and KSU Speech Discrimination (Berger, 1969). All these materials are developed with multiple lists which are supposedly equivalent and which can be used to assess the ability of youngsters to perform using the modalities described above. For more information on both word lists and sentences, the reader is referred to Olsen and Matkin (1979).

Comprehension of Spoken Language

The key to this section is comprehension. The section above was concerned only with the ability to receive information. Brackett (1982) subdivided this area into 3 categories: single-word receptive vocabulary, morphology and syntax, and paragraph comprehension. The assessment of single-word receptive vocabulary can be accomplished through a variety of tests such as the Peabody Picture Vocabulary Test (PPVT) (Dunn & Dunn, 1981), the Test of Language Development (TOLD) (Newcomer & Hammill, 1982), or the

Boehm Test of Basic Concepts (Boehm, 1971). Morphology and syntax might be assessed through such measures as the Test of Auditory Comprehension of Language (TACL) (Carrow, 1973), the Northwestern Syntax Screening Test (NSST) (Lee, 1971), and the Test of Syntactic Abilities (TSA) (Quigley, Stein- kamp, Power, & Jones, 1978). Reynell Developmental Language Scale: Verbal Comprehension Scale (Reynell, 1977) and the Miller Yoder Test of Grammat- ical Comprehension (Miller & Yoder, 1975). The assessment of paragraph comprehension might be assessed with such tests as the Durrell Paragraph Listening Test (Durrell, 1955), the Test of Auditory Comprehension (TAC) (Audiologic Services & Southwest School for the Hearing Impaired, 1976) or the Clinical Evaluation of Language Function (Semel & Wiig, 1980).

Production of Spoken Language

The assessment of a youngster's ability to use spoken language should be assessed on the basis of morphology and syntax and the use of language. Brackett (1982) suggests that morphology and snytax be assessed using the Developmental Sentence Analysis (DSA) (Lee, 1974), a Spontaneous Lan- guage Analysis System outlined by Kretschmer and Kretschmer (1978), an elicited language sample modeled after the approach suggested by the Gram- matical Evaluation of Language (GAEL) (Moog & Geers, 1979), or the Carrow Elicited Language Inventory (CELI) (Carrow-Woolfolk, 1974).

The use of language can be assessed by dividing this area into 2 subareas: lexical use and connected speech. There are a number of possible tests to evaluate the lexicon of a youngster. The Wechsler Intelligence Scale for Chil- dren—Revised (WISC-R) (Wechsler, 1974) vocabulary subtest would be ap- propriate. The Test of Language Development (TOLD) (Newcomer & Ham- mill, 1982) oral vocabulary subtest could be also be used. The Detroit Test of Learning Aptitude (Baker & Bernice, 1967) verbal opposites and likenessess and differences subtests would also measure lexical aspects of spoken lan- guage. The Oral Vocabulary subtest of the TOLD or the picture vocabulary subtest of the Woodcock-Johnson Psycho-Education Battery (Woodcock & Johnson, 1977) could also be used, as could the Oral Vocabulary and gram- mar completion subtest of the TOLD. Connected speech could be assessed using the Detroit Test of Learning Aptitude (Hammill, 1984) verbal absurdities and social adjustment subtest, as well as information and comprehension subtests from the WISC-R.

Production of Speech

For evaluating the production of speech, it is recommended that 3 levels be assessed: sound and syllable level, word level, and speech intelligibility. These can be assessed by using the Ling Phonetic Level Evaluation, pp. 150– 168 (Ling, 1976) for syllables, an articulation test for the assessement of words, and the NTID Rating Scale (Johnson, 1976) to obtain a measure of an individual's speech intelligibility. Another test suggested by Moeller, McConkey, and Osberger (1983) is the Speech-Intelligibility Evaluation (SPINE). Chapter 6 also addresses this area of assessment.

Comprehension and Production of Written Language

For evaluating the comprehension of written syntax, one test to be used in the Test of Syntactic Ability Screening Test (Quigley, Steinkamp, Power, & Jones, 1978). The evaluation of written language is accomplished through the use of an elicited or spontaneous language sample of perhaps the Picture Story Language Test (Myklebust, 1965), although this particular test must be restandardized and updated to reflect current knowledge of language.

Communicative Competence

Finally, the ability of the hearing-impaired youngster to use language communicatively needs to be evaluated. Brackett (1983) divides this into 2 areas: the function of language and the style of language use. The function of language is assessed by determining if youngsters know how to sustain a topic of conversation, use flexible language, demonstrate both polite and authoritarian routines, and adapt the message after a communication failure or upon the listener's request. The style of language is assessed by determining youngsters' awareness of a listener's knowledge and status and appropriate adaptation of the message. Additionally, individuals need to understand and use conversational turn-taking strategies and to observe appropriate entry points.

Moeller (1984) and Vernon, McConkey, & Osberger (1983) add a few ideas to those suggested above. First, it is critical to realize that formal testing needs to be augmented by informal tests and diagnostic teaching if one is to understand the extent of problems hearing-impaired youngsters are experiencing. Moeller also suggests that thought-related language skills are important to assess. She suggests that the Test of Concept Utilization (Crager & Springs, 1972) and the Test of Problem Solving (Fachman, Jorgensen, Husingh, & Barrett, 1984) are appropriate tests to use in the assessment of thinking with language and of problem solving.

Moeller (1984) also suggests that question comprehension of the hearing impaired is important to assess. Russell, Quigley, & Power, pp. 126–127 (1976) have found that the hearing impaired have considerable difficulty in the area of question usage. Moeller suggests that the use of the Preschool Language Assessment Instrument (Blanck, Rose, & Berlin 1978) and Classroom Questions Test (Sanders, 1966) are effective tools in measuring question forms. Through careful analysis, it is possible to learn not only the kinds of questions that are problematical but also the thinking process that is tapped by the questions forms.

Finally, Moeller (1984) suggests that youngsters need to be assessed in their classrooms, under normal conditions. This is really an informal assessment of youngsters as the assessor observes them engaging in interactive discourse with the teachers and peers in a normal classroom setting. By observing youngsters under these conditions, it is possible to obtain a basic idea of the strengths and weaknesses students have in real situations rather than under the strained and formal conditions present in a testing situation.

ADAPTIVE SKILLS OR SOCIAL MATURITY

The fifth and final area in the PEMICS model is social maturity. One of the primary functions in the assessment process is to determine how well an individual is able to function in society. It seems to the authors that the primary goal of education is to help individuals obtain a certain level of independence so that they can work, live, and enjoy a happy, independent, and productive life. One method of trying to assess this ability is through the use of measures of adaptive abilities. The assessment of adaptive behavior is, however, somewhat different than the measurement of other functions previously discussed. Ordinarily, the individual being assessed is asked to perform some task that is scored and the performance is compared to that of a sample population or some other criterion. In measuring adaptive behaviors, a third person, who is very familiar with the subject under study, is interviewed. The assessor interviews the third person, who is invited to describe the behavior patterns of the subject.

There are a number of devices available for the measure of adaptive skills, however, there is only one measure that has been used with the hearing impaired to any significant extent: the Vineland Social Maturity Scale (Doll, 1965). The Vineland is arranged into eight clusters of social competence across the age span from birth to 30 years of age. This tremendous age span indicates the wide variability of items sampled. The following list provides the reader with a basic idea of the areas evaluated.

Self-Help General. The items under this general heading sample activities such as sitting, standing, caring for oneself at the toilet, and avoiding simple hazards.

Self-Help Eating. The items under this general heading are focused on individuals' abilities to care for themselves at the table while eating. It begins with items such as drinking from a cup with assistance and progresses to the point where youngsters are cutting their own meat unassisted.

Self-Help Dressing. The items under this general heading assess individuals' increasing independence in dressing and personal hygiene. The items assess progress from issues like buttoning to the complete care for and maintenance of clothing.

Locomotion. The items under this heading address the individual's ability to move around in the environment. This area samples such skills as walking and progresses to items like going to near or distant places unattended.

Occupation. The items in this area examine issues beginning with youngsters' abilities to occupy themselves while unattended, progressing up to the ability to perform expert work and engage in beneficial recreation.

Communication. The items under this heading examine the ability of subjects to engage in increasingly demanding forms of communication. This area samples such issues as being able to imitate speech and progresses up to the ability to read, write, and use the telephone. Obviously, hearing-impaired individuals will score below normal in this area, not because of low social adaptation skills, but because of the breakdown in the ability to communicate due to language and hearing problems.

Self-Direction. The issues evaluated here are things like the ability to use money and the ability to assume responsiblity for oneself. This area thus assesses issues such as being trusted with money and progresses to the ability to buy all of one's own clothing. This area also focuses on issues such as youngsters' ability to go into the neighborhood unattended or individuals' looking after their own health.

Socialization. The issues under this area focus on individuals' interpersonal relations. Some of the items assessed are playing games effectively with other people and promoting the general welfare of society at large.

As can be seen, the area of social adaptation is very large and quite unique. As suggested earlier in the chapter, part of the purpose of the case history interview is to obtain information that can be evaluated by the use of a social adaptation scale.

There is a new Vineland Adaptive Behavior Scale (Sparrow, Balla, & Cicchetti, 1984) that may prove a useful tool in the assessment of adaptive abilities, especially since the Vineland Scale of Social Maturity is somewhat suspect due to the normative sample and the changes that have occurred in society since 1957.

Vocational Interests.   Another area that falls under the general area of social maturity is vocational interests. Although there are a number of post-secondary programs available to the hearing impaired, the average hearing-impaired individual ends formal schooling at the end of high school or before. This suggests that educators need to be concerned that hearing-impaired youngsters, upon completion of high school, have some skills that can be used in the workplace and in living generally. As in other areas examined, there are not a large number of tools avilable to use in assessing the hearing impaired. Zieziula, Chapter 7 (1982) does report that there are some tests that can be used, if used carefully.

A study completed by Hanrahan (1983) found that two of the vocational interest surveys he used were not very helpful as standardized tests, but rather he indicated that these tests can be used as a means of finding out about some interests and in helping educators develop vocational interests in hearing-impaired individuals. In other words, the tests should be given as early as possible in the adolescent years as a means of determining general areas of interest and as a precursor to educating youngsters about the job market, with the aim of helping to give them direction in the selection of a job that will have the potential of providing satisfaction in the workplace.

Synthesis and Evaluation of Data

The global assessment described above is intended to help parents, school, and habilitative specialists understand the hearing-impaired youngster's strengths, weaknesses, and general abilities to perform tasks, and to understand the strategies that might be used to help such a youngster achieve maximal growth. By using the information obtained from parental input, direct observation of youngsters, and the results of tests, it will be possible to provide appropriate services to individuals. The nature of the help, of course, depends on the needs of the individual. It seems to the authors, however, that once a complete picture is obtained, it is critical that there be professionals in the educational system who will take an active part in assuring, as much as possible, that the recommendations are in fact carried out, and that youngsters are reevaluated on a periodic basis to be certain that individual needs are being met. It may not be necessary to do the in-depth evaluation described in this chapter for every hearing-impaired child with loses ranging from slight to profound. It seems, however, that in order to provide help to all children, it is necessary to screen children not only in terms of audition, but in a global manner. When there is reason to believe that youngsters have additional problems beyond hearing loss, then additional testing should be recommended. Chapter 8 addresses the overall management of the hearing impaired.

Case Study

Table 3-1 illustrates the result of a global evaluation of D.C., a young hearing-impaired boy who was seen for a comprehensive evaluation when he was 10 years of age. According to the case history interview, both birth history and developmental history were normal. Health history was normal, indicating minimal problems during early childhood and no history of significant middle ear disease. Parents became concerned with the child's hearing after D's first birthday. When visiting their pediatrician, however, they were told not to be concerned. At 18 months, the parents were still concerned with hearing and sought a second opinion. They were referred to an audiologist for a complete

Table 3-1.
Profile of D.C., age 10 years 0 months

Stanine	1	2	3	4	5	6	7	8	9
Vision									
20/200 without correction			*						
20/20 corrected					*				
eye teaming					*				
binocularity					*				
visual perception					*				
visual-motor					*				
Emotion			*						
Motor									
gross motor									
running speed					*				
balance		*							
bilateral coordination			*						
fine motor									
response speed					*				
visual motor control				*					
Intelligence									
verbal			*						
performance									
WISC-R					*				
Hiskey-Nebraska				*					
Learning Abilities									
visual memory			*						
auditory memory		*							
part-whole relationships							*		
Language									
vocabulary (receptive)		*							
vocabulary (expressive)	*								
syntax (written)				*					
written language (general)		*							
reading									
comprehension		*							
mechanics					*				
math (language problems)		*							
math (computation)					*				
Social Maturity					*				

audiological evaluation. The audiological evaluation revealed a severe, bilateral sensori-neural hearing loss. D.C. was fitted with 2 binaural hearing aids at age two and began receiving language training in the home. Shortly after his second birthday, D. uttered his first recognizable word.

At age three, D. was enrolled in a preschool program for the hearing impaired, where he continued until he turned 8 years of age. For the past 2 years, he has been enrolled in regular elementary school classrooms for all but 2 hours of the day. During these 2 hours, he receives remedial help from a teacher of the hearing impaired in reading and language.

Both the regular classroom teacher and the teacher of the hearing impaired report that D. frequently becomes angry when he is asked to perform tasks that he believes to be too difficult. When angry, he will throw objects (such as books) around the classroom and refuse to do any work. Both parents report that D. is occasionally difficult to manage at home. Mrs. C. reports that her husband has a violent temper and that family arguments are common.

Behavior during the assessment revealed a youngster who was basically cooperative, but who needed considerable encouragement. D. asked that instructions be repeated and often asked if he could repeat a task to be sure that he "got it right." He was only marginally interested in most of the tasks that were attempted, and he appeared to lose interest in tasks quickly; as items became more difficult, he began to fidget in his chair a great deal. As the test items reached levels beyond his ability, he would exhibit some avoidance behaviors, such as saying that he had forgotten how to do the assigned task, or couldn't remember, or needed to sharpen his pencil, or ask if we were almost finished.

Perceptual Testing. Audiological findings revealed a severe sensori-neural loss in the right ear and a severe-to-profound sensori-neural loss in the left ear with pure-tone averages of 65 dB in the right ear and 92 dB in the left. Speech Reception Thresholds of 66 dB for the right and 90 dB for the left ear were in excellent agreement with the pure-tone averages. Speech discrimination scores of 80 percent were obtained by presenting phonetically balanced kindergarten (PB-K) word lists at a level of +40 sensation level (SL) in the right ear, using a monitored live voice technique. No speech recognition score was obtained beyond the speech reception threshold (SRT) in the left ear; he was only able to understand highly redundant, very familiar words in the left ear. Impedance testing was normal bilaterally.

His speech reception threshold was assessed with his behind-the-ear Oticon hearing aids. While wearing both aids, an SRT of 45 dB was obtained. The SRT was retested with an aid in his right ear only and a threshold of 25 dB was obtained. D's ability to repeat monosyllabic words with both aids on at 50 dBHL was then measured using PB-K materials and a score of 50 percent was obtained. He was then retested with one aid in the right ear and he obtained a score of 80 percent. This finding suggests that D. may perform significantly better with one aid. D. was then retested with one hearing aid in a background of noise and it was found that his discrimination score dropped to 65 percent. When he was tested again with 2 aids in the background of noise, his discrimination score decreased to 25 percent. These findings confirm that D. seems to perform best with one aid in his right ear, and, if the listening environment is very quiet, he performs significantly better. Finally, when speech materials were presented to D. using both auditory and visual input in a background of noise, his repetition scores improved to 95 percent, suggesting that D. needs to be in a position to see the speaker in order to obtain maximum information.

Visually, D. performed within normal limits when wearing his corrective lenses: eye teaming, binocularity, near and far seeing abilities, as well as visual perception and visual motor skills, were all within normal limits.

Emotional/Psycho-Social Skills. D. was found to be cooperative in a structured situation, yet defensive. He performed the assigned tasks, but he did not relate well to the examiner directly. He was rigid and concrete in all that he did, performing in a very mechanistic way. In contrast, in the unstructured situation he did relate in a more relaxed fashion. He initiated some direct interaction and seemed to feel much less threatened. His drawings seem to indicate that he is insecure, rigid, sensitive to criticism, overdefensive, and hostile to those whom he perceives as being a threat to him. He demonstrates fear of interpersonal relationships and a basic anxiety over his own intellectual abilities. He loses control of his impulses at times. He appears to feel that his body and mind are separate entities and act independently from each other unexpectedly. He compensates for feelings of lack of control by becoming overcontrolled. He tends to structure the environment in such a way as to keep conscious control over everything around him.

Motor. Performance on the Bruininks-Oseretsky Test of Motor Proficiency indicated that in the area of gross motor abilities, he was within the normal range for running speed and agility, but significantly below normal in general balance and bilateral coordination. In the area of fine motor development, he scored within the normal range. Given the low scores in the gross motor area, an Occupational Therapist needs to be consulted to do a more complete assessment.

Intelligence. Performance on the WISC-R placed D in the low average of general abilities. There was a significant difference between his functioning in verbal and visual testing in most areas. D's learning age on the Hiskey-Nebraska Test of Learning Aptitude was also within the normal range, confirming the finding that D's general cognitive abilities are normal. There were some findings on the intelligence test that suggest possible areas of strengths and weakness.

Learning Abilities. Testing in learning areas suggested some specific areas of strength and weakness that could not be accounted for on the basis of hearing loss alone. The scores D. obtained on the vocabulary subtest of the WISC-R were significantly below the other verbal scores. Additionally, the score obtained on the coding subtest was significantly below the other performance scores. On selected subtests from the Detroit Test of Learning Aptitude and the Hiskey-Nebraska Test of Learning Aptitude, D. had difficulty with tasks requiring memory, such as the Information subtest, Auditory Attention for both unrelated and related words and syllables, and Memory for Color. His greatest difficulty appears to be auditory memory tasks, particularly when memory of syllables and words is involved. He also has some difficulty with visual memory tasks when the materials are nonmeaningful and when there is little opportunity for an auditory mediation.

D. appears to have considerable strength in being able to see part-whole relationships. He appears to be able to visually identify essential parts and to see the relations of parts to one another.

Academic Achievement/Communication. Academically, D.C. generally performs at a third grade level. His abilities in reading mechanics appear to be appropriate to his age in work knowledge, although comprehension of what he reads is significantly below his grade placement. He demonstrated excellent ability to pronounce and analyze words. In mathematical problem solving, he scored at a level appropriate to his grade placement. In sharp contrast, when language was necessary to solve problems, he scored significantly below his grade level, having the most difficulty with word problems and measurements, i.e., differentiating inches, yards, feet, meters, and centimeters. D's written response to a standardized picture consisted of simple sentences following a basic pattern of subject-verb-object. His writing was very concrete and consisted of many carrier phrases, i.e.: "The boy sat by the table." "The boy pushed the doll," etc. He made no syntactic errors, but did make a few morphological errors. In most aspects, the story was like that which a 7- or 8- year-old boy might write. His spelling was considerably better than expected; he obtained a score appropriate to his chronological age. He demonstrated excellent word analysis and phonic skills, which was surprising given the degree of his hearing impairment.

Social Maturity. In the area of social maturity, D. scored at a level appropriate to his chronological age, suggesting that his overall maturity is good. Had the items that were not scoreable (mostly due to communication problems related to his hearing loss) been scored as acceptable, his scores would have improved to that of a youngster 10 years and 9 months of age.

Summary and Recommendations. D.C. is a 10-year-old male with a moderate-to-severe sensori-neural loss in the right ear and a severe to profound sensori-neural hearing loss in the left ear. He appears to function best with one aid fitted to the right ear in a quiet environment. This youngster has additional problems in reading comprehension which may be related to visual and auditory memory abilities. D. appears to have normal intelligence and has been able to make good use of visual information to offset, to some extent, the effects imposed by his auditory impairments. It also appears that D. is having some emotional difficulties. Finally, D. may have some motor difficulties which need to be given attention. In view of these findings, the following recommendations were made:

1. D. should continue to be evaluated in a diagnostic teaching environment to determine the exact nature of his reading difficulty and to discover the best teaching techniques to be used in remediating this difficulty.
2. An in-depth psychological assessment and parent interview need to be conducted in order to determine the need for individual or perhaps family counseling.
3. D. needs to have continued placement with a teacher of the hearing impaired at least for part of the academic day in order to receive continued help in language and vocabulary development. It may be necessary, however, to attempt some learning strategies that use visual, auditory, and tactile modes in order to help him remember better.
4. It is critical that he be in a quiet setting where he can see and hear the instructor. It might be very helpful for D. to use a frequency modulation (FM) system for instructional periods.
5. The academic activities in the regular classroom must be carefully coordinated with the activities in the resource classroom or other settings if there is to be meaningful transfer from one learning environment to another. Too much fragmentation in learning will only lead to confusion.

REFERENCES

Alexander J. Ocular abnormalities among congenitally deaf children. *Canadian Journal of Ophthalmology,* 1973, 8, pp. 175–189.

Allen W. Vision screening programs for hearing impaired children and youth. Paper presented at the International Convention of the Alexander Graham Bell Association for the Deaf, Houston, Texas, June, 1980.

Arthur G. *Arthur adaptation of the Leiter International Performance Scale.* Los Angeles: Western Psychological Services, 1950.

Audiologic Services & Southwest School for the Hearing Impaired, *Test of auditory comprehension.* North Hollywood, California: Foreworks, 1976.

Ayres J. *Sensory integration and learning disorders.* Los Angeles: Western Psychological Services, 1972.

Bannatyne, A. *Language, reading and learning disabilities,* Springfield, Illinois: Charles C. Thomas, 1971, p. 98.

Baker J, & Bernice L. *Detroit Test of Learning Aptitude.* Indianapolis: Bobbs-Merrill Co., 1967.

Battin R. Psycho-educational assessment of children with auditory language learning problems. In R Roeser, & M Downs, (Eds.), *Auditory disorders in school children.* New York: Thieme-Stratton, 1981.

Beery, K E, & Buktenica, N. *Developmental Test of Visual-Motor Integration.* Chicago: Follet, 1967.

Berger K. Speech discrimination task using multiple choice key words in sentences. *Journal of Auditory Research,* 1969, *9,* 247–262.

Billar C. Signs of gross and fine motor difficulties. Lecture in Com D 639, Logan, Utah: Utah State University, Spring, 1983.

Blair J. *The contributing influences of amplification, speechreading and classroom environments on the ability of hard-of-hearing children to discriminate sentences.* Unpublished doctoral dissertation, Northwestern University, 1976.

Blair J. Unpublished research, Logan, Utah: Utah State University, 1983

Blair J. Peterson M. & Viehweg S. The effects of mild hearing loss on academic performance among school-age children. The Volta Review, 1985, 87-94

Blair, J, Wright K, & Pollard G. Parental understanding of their children's hearing aids. *Volta Review,* 1981, *83,* 375–382.

Blank M, Rose S, & Berlin L. *Preschool language assessment Instrument.* New York: Grune & Stratton, 1978.

Bloom B (Ed.). *Taxonomy of educational objectives: The classification of educational goals, Handbook 2, Cognitive domain.* New York: McKay, 1956, p. 10.

Bloom B, Hastings J, & Madaus G. *Handbook of formative and summative evaluation of student learning.* New York: McGraw-Hill, 1971, p. 37.

Boehm A. Boehm test of basic concepts. New York: The Psychological Corporation, 1971.

Brackett D. Language assessment protocols for hearing-impaired students. *Topics in Language Disorders.* June 1982, pp. 46–56.

Bricklin B, Zygmunt P, & Wagner E. *The Hand Test* (6th printing). Springfield, Illinois: Charles C. Thomas, 1981.

Brown A, Stein S, & Rohrer P. *The Chicago Non-Verbal Examination.* New York: Psychological Corporation, 1947.

Bruininks, R. *Bruininks-Oseretsky test of motor proficiency.* Circle Pines, Minnesota, 1978.

Buck J & Jolles I. *House-Tree-Person.* Los Angeles: Western Psychological Services, 1966.

Burks H. *Burks Behavior Rating Scales: Manual.* Los Angeles: Western Psychological Services, 1977.

Carrow E. *Test for auditory comprehension of language.* Austin, Texas: Learning Concepts, 1973.

Carrow-Wolfolk E. *Carrow elicited language inventory.* Austin, Texas: Learning Concepts, 1974.

Chandler T. Locus of control: A proposal for change. *Psychology in the Schools,* 1975, *12,* 335–339.

Clark T, & Watkins S. *The Ski*Hi model, programming for hearing impaired infants through home intervention, home visit curriculum* (4th ed.), 31–55. Logan, Utah: Ski*Hi Institute, 1985.

Coan R, & Cattell R. *Early School Personality Questionnaire.* Champaign, Il: Institute for Personality and Ability Testing, 1976.

Cohen R. Auditory skills and the communicative process. In R. Keith (Ed.), *Seminars in speech, language and hearing.* New York: Thieme-Stratton, 1980.

Colarusso R & Hammill D. *Motor-Free Visual Perception Test.* Novato: Academic Therapy Publications, 1972.

Cole P & Wood ML Differential Diagnosis. In F Martin (Ed.) *Pediatric audiology,* New Jersey; Prentice-Hall, 1978.

Crager R & Springs A. *The Test of Concept Utilization*. Los Angeles: Western Psychological Association, 1972.

Doll E. *Vineland Social Maturity Scale*. Circle Pines, Mn: Educational Testing Service, 1965.

Dunn L & Dunn L. *Peabody Picture Vocabulary Test-Revised*. Circle Pines, MN: American Guidance Service, 1981.

Durrell D. *Durrell analysis of reading difficulty*. New York: Harcourt Brace Jovanovich, Publishers, 1955.

Elliott L & Katz D. *Northwestern University Children's Perception of Speech (NU-CHIPS)*. St. Louis: Auditec of St. Louis, 1980.

Fachman L, Jorgensen C, Husingh R, & Barrett M. *Test of Problem Solving*. Moline, Ill: Linguisystems, 1984.

Farnsworth D. *The Farnsworth Dichotomous Test For Color Blindness*. Cleveland: The Psychological Corporation, 1947.

Frankenburg W & Dodds J. *Denver Developmental Screening Test* (rev.). Denver: University of Colorado Medical Center, 1970.

Fuller C. The case history interview. In F Berg & S Fletcher (Eds.), *The hard of hearing child*. New York: Grune & Stratton, 1970, pp. 191–202.

Goodenough F & Harris D. *Goodenough-Harris Drawing Test*. Los Angeles: Western Psychological Services, 1963.

Hammill D. *Detroit Test of Learning Aptitude, 1984 Revision (DTLA-2)*. Los Angeles: Western Psychological Services, 1984.

Hanrahan P. *Measurement of the career interests of hearing-impaired students in regular high schools*. Unpublished masters thesis, Utah State University, 1983.

Hardy LH, Rand G, & Ritter M. *AOH-R-R pseudoisochromatic plates*. Buffalo: American Optical Co. Instrument Division, 1957.

Haskins H. *A Phonetically Balanced Test of Speech Discrimination for Children*. Unpublished masters thesis. Northwestern University, 1949.

Hirsh F, Davis H, Silverman S, Reynolds E. Eldert E, & Benson R. Development of materials for speech audiometry. *Journal of Speech and Hearing Disorders*, 1952, *17*, 321–337.

Hiskey M. *Hiskey-Nebraska Test of Learning Aptitude*. Lincoln, Neb: Marshall S. Hiskey, 1966.

Ishihara S. *Ishihara Color Blind Test Book (Children)*. Tokyo: Kanehara Shuppan, 1970.

Johnson D. Communication characteristics of a young deaf adult population: Techniques for evaluating their communication skills. *American Annals of the Deaf*, August 1976, pp. 409–424.

Kalikow D & Stevens, K. Development of a test of speech intelligibility in noise using sentence materials with controlled word predictability. *Journal of the Acoustical Society of America*, 1977, *61*, 5.

Keith R. *Central auditory dysfunction*. New York: Grune & Stratton, 1977.

Keith R. Tests of central auditory function. In R Roeser & M Downs (Eds.), *Auditory disorders in school children*. New York: Thieme-Stratton, 1981, pp. 164–167.

Kretschmer R & Kretschmer L. *Language development and intervention with the hearing-impaired*. Baltimore: University Park Press, 1978.

Kretschmer R & Quigley S. The psycho-educational assessment of hearing-impaired children. In R Roeser & M Downs (Eds.), *Auditory disorders in school children*. New York: Thieme-Stratton, 1981, p. 208.

Kübler-Ross E. *On death and dying*. New York: Macmillan, 1969.

Lee L. *Developmental sentence analysis*. Evanston, Illinois: Northwestern University Press, 1974.

Lee L. *Northwestern syntax screening test*. Evanston, Illinois: Northwestern University Press, 1971.

Leiter R. *Leiter International Performance Scale*. Los Angeles: Western Psychological Services, 1949.

Levine E. Psycho-social determinants in personality development. *Volta Review*, 1976, *78*, 258-267.

Levine E & Wagner E. Personality patterns of deaf persons: An interpretation based on research with the hand test. *Perceptual Motor Skills,* 1974, 39, 1167-1236.

Ling D. *Speech and hearing impaired child: Theory and practice.* Washington, D.C.: Alexander Graham Bell Association for the Deaf, 1976.

Luterman D. *Counseling parents of hearing-impaired children.* Boston: Little Brown, 1979.

Matkin N, Hook P & Hixson, P. A multidisciplinary approach to the evaluation of hearing-impaired children. In L Bradford & F Martin, (Eds.), *Audiology, an audio journal for continuing education, Volume 4, Number 7,* 1979.

Maxon A, Brackett D, & van den Berg S. Socialization of the mainstreamed hearing impaired child. Poster session presented at the Alexander Graham Bell Association Conference, Toronto, June, 1982.

McCrone W. Learned helplessness and level of underachievement among deaf adolescents. *Psychology in the Schools,* 1979, *16,* 430; 434

Miller J & Yoder D. *Miller-Yoder test of grammatical comprehension.* Madison, Wisconsin: University of Wisconsin, unpublished experimental edition, 1975.

Miller L. *Louisville Behavior Checklist: Manual.* Los Angeles: Western Psychological Services, 1977.

Moeller M P. The hard-of-hearing, school-aged child: Evaluation and remediation issues. Michigan: Van Riper Lecture Series, September, 1984.

Moeller M P, McConkey A, & Osberger M J. Evaluation of the communicative skills of hearing-impaired children. *Audiology,* August 1983, pp. 113–127.

Moeller M P, Osberger M J, McConkey A, & Eccarius M. Some language skills of the student in a residential school for the deaf. *Journal of the Academy of Rehabilitative Audiology,* 1981, 14, 84–111.

Mohindra I. Vision profile of deaf children. *American Journal of Optometry and Physiological Optics,* 1976, *53,* 126–143.

Moog J, & Geers A. *CID Grammatical Analysis of Elicited Language.* St. Louis, MO: Central Institute for the Deaf, 1979.

Moores D. *Educating the deaf, psychology, principles and practices.* Boston: Houghton Mifflin, 1978.

Moses K. Observation of children in a psychological assessment. Class notes for D-49, Introduction to Counseling for the Hearing Impaired, Northwestern University, Winter, 1973.

Moses K. Parenting a hearing impaired child. *Volta Review,* Feb/Mar., 1979, 73–80

Murray H, *Thematic Apperception Test.* Cambridge, Mass: Harvard University Press, 1943.

Myklebust H. *Auditory disorder in children.* New York: Grune & Stratton, 1954.

Myklebust H. *Development and disorders of written language. Volume one, Picture story language test.* New York: Grune & Stratton, 1965, pp. 36–44.

Myklebust H. *Psychology of deafness.* New York: Grune & Stratton, 1960, p. 184.

National Commission on Excellence in Education. *A nation at risk: The imperative for educational reform.* Secretary of Education, United States Department of Education, April, 1983.

Newcomer P & Hammill D. *Test of language development.* Monterey, California: Publishers: Test Service, 1982.

Northern J & Downs M. *Hearing in children* (3rd ed.) Baltimore: Williams & Wilkins, 1984.

Olsen W & Matkin N. Speech audiometry. In W. Rintelmann (Ed.) *Hearing assessment,* Baltimore: University Park Press, 1979.

Patterson E & Williams J. Intelligence of deaf children as measured by drawings. *American Annals of the Deaf,* 1930 75, 273–290.

Pollard G & Neumaier R. Vision characteristics of deaf students. *American Annals of the deaf,* December, 1974, pp. 740–745.

Quigley S & Kretschmer R. *The education of deaf children, issues, theory and practice.* Baltimore: University Park Press, 1982.

Quigley S, Steinkamp M, Powers: D, & Jones B. *Test of syntactic abilities.* Beaverton, Oregon: Dormac, Inc. 1978.

Quigley S & Paul P. *Language and deafness.* San Diego: College-Hill Press, 1984, pp. 49–64

Rainer J & Altshuler K. *Psychiatry and the deaf, workshop for the psychiatrist.* New York State Psychiatric Institute, 1967.

Raven J C, Court J H, & Raven J. *Standard progressive matrices.* London: H.K. Lewis & Co. Ltd., 1977.

Reynell S. *Reynell developmental language scale.* Windsor, England: NFER Publishing, 1977.

Rorschach H. *Rorschach ink blot test.* New York: Grune & Stratton, 1966.

Rosenberg P. Case history: The first test. In J. Katz. (Ed.) *Handbook of clinical audiology,* (2nd Ed.), Baltimore: Williams and Wilkins, 1978.

Ross M. with Brackett D, & Maxon A. *Hard of hearing children in regular schools.* New Jersey: Prentice-Hall, 1982.

Ross M & Lerman J. *Word intelligibility by picture identification.* Pittsburg: Stanwix House, 1971, p. 102.

Rotter J. Generalized expectancies for internal versus external control of reinforcement. *Psychological Monographs,* 1966, *80,* 534–544.

Rules and Regulations of the Education of All Handicapped Children Act of 1975. U.S. Dept. of Health, Education and Welfare, 1977, Federal Register 42, 42474-42518.

Russell W K, Quigley S P, & Power D J. *Linguistics and deaf children.* Washington, D.C.: Alexander Graham Bell Association for the Deaf, 1976.

Salvia J & Ysseldyke J. *Assessment in special and remedial education,* (3rd ed.). Boston: Houghton Mifflin, 1985, p. 99, 126–127, 138, 217, 220

Sanders, N M. *Classroom questions—what kinds?* New York: Harper & Row, 1966.

Schlesinger H & Meadow K. *Sound and sign.* Berkeley: University of California Press, 1972.

Semel E & Wiig E. *Clinical evaluation of language functions.* Columbus, Ohio: Charles E. Merrill Co., 1980.

Shephard N, Davis J, Gorga M, & Stelmachowicz P. Characteristics of hearing impaired children in the public schools: Part I—Demographic data. *Journal of Speech and Hearing Disorders,* 1981, *46,* 123–129.

Silverman S & Hirsh I. Problems related to the use of speech in clinical audiometry. *Annals of Otology Rhinology Laryngology,* 1955, *64;* 1234–1244.

Smith, P. *Perceptual Motor Test.* New York: Educational Activities, Inc., 1967.

Sparrow S, Balla D, & Cicchetti D. *Vineland Adaptive Scales.* Circle Pines MN. American Guidance Service, 1984.

Suchman E. Visual defects in the deaf child. *Archives of Ophthalmology,* 1967, 67(18), 127–140.

Sussman A & Stewart L. *Counseling with deaf people.* New York: Deafness Research and Training Center, New York University School of Education, 1971.

Urban W. *Draw-A-Person Projective Technique.* Los Angeles: Western Psychological Services, 1963.

Vernon, M. Sociological & psychological factors associated with hearing loss. *Journal of Speech & Hearing Research,* 1969, *12,* 541–563.

Vernon M P, McConkey A, & Osberger M J. Evaluation of the communicative skills of hearing-impaired children. *Audiology,* August 1983, pp. 113–127.

Wagner E. *The Hand Test, Revised.* Los Angeles: Western Psychological Services, 1983.

Waller N, Sollad R, Sander E, & Kunicki E. Psychological assessment of speech and language-disordered children. *Language, Speech, and Hearing Services in Schools,* April 1983, pp. 92–98.

Watkins S. *Longitudinal study of the effects of home intervention on hearing impaired children.* Unpublished doctoral dissertation. Utah State University, 1984.

Weber S & Reddell R. A sentence test for measuring speech discrimination in children. *Audiology Hearing and Education.* 1976, 2(25), 30–40.

Wechsler D. *Manual for the Wechsler Preschool and Primary Scale of Intelligence.* Cleveland: The Psychological Corporation, 1967.

Wechsler D. *Manual for the Wechsler Intelligence Scale for Children-Revised.* Cleveland: The Psychological Corporation, 1974.

Wechsler D. *Manual for the Wechsler Adult Intelligence Scale-Revised.* New York: Psychological Corporation, 1981.

Woodcock R & Johnson M. *Woodcock-Johnson psychoeducational battery.* Boston: Teaching Resources, 1977.

Wyatt G. *Language learning and communication disorders in children.* New York: Free Press, 1969.

Zieziula F. (Ed.). *Assessment of hearing-impaired people, a guide for selecting psychological, educational and vocational tests.* Washington, D.C.: Gallaudet College Press, 1982, p. 83.

Steven H. Veihweg

4
Audiological Considerations

To a large extent, the effect of hearing loss on various aspects of development is dependent on the magnitude and configuration of the hearing loss. An audiological evaluation must be performed in order to secure data related to magnitude of hearing loss and audiometric configuration. Typically, a basic comprehensive audiological evaluation consists of pure-tone air and bone-conduction thresholds, speech reception thresholds, and speech discrimination scores. Some audiologists include such acoustic immittance measures as typanometry, static compliance, and acoustic reflex thresholds as part of the basic comprehensive audiological evaluation. Together with the case history information, data from these tests serve as the springboard for making many audiological, educational, and medical decisions. Decisions as to what additional special audiological tests to administer are based largely on information obtained from the case history and from the basic comprehensive audiological evaluation, as are decisions regarding need for amplification, need for medical referral, need for educational/psychological testing, and need for speech and language evaluation and intervention.

Before a basic comprehensive audiological evaluation is conducted, there is usually a perceived need. The perceived need may originate from any of several sources, including parents and/or other significant persons, teachers, other educators, and the child. Often, however, mild hearing loss (and sometimes moderate hearing loss) goes undetected in school-age children until a hearing screening test is conducted in conjunction with the educational programs of the school. Several different protocols for hearing screening have been proposed across the years and, although all have factors to recommend their use, some methods and procedures seem to be considerably more successful in identifying children with potential hearing problems than are others.

The goal of the present chapter is to present current principles, practices, and philosophies associated with identification audiometry and to discuss the major tests and materials used in diagnostic audiological evaluation of school-age children.

IDENTIFICATION AUDIOMETRY

In years gone by, the single component involved in public school hearing screening testing has been pure-tone air-conduction sweep frequency screening. Data existent since the 1960s (Eagles, Wishik, Doerfler, Melnick, & Levine, 1963) indicate that pure-tone air-conduction sweep frequency testing using a level of 20 or 25 dB HL will fail to identify approximately 50 percent of children with active middle ear disease at the time of the screening. Consequently, there has been a great need to revise and upgrade screening procedures in order to identify a greater proportion of children with active middle ear disease who have fluctuating hearing loss and pure-tone thresholds better than 25 dB HL. In recent years, 2 factors have made it possible to greatly improve the results of public school hearing screening programs. First, audiologists have become less reluctant to look inside ears in performing a very elementary and rudimentary otoscopic examination and, second, immittance instrumentation has become available at a price affordable for many school districts. It is to be hoped that hearing screening programs of the future will incorporate all 3 components namely: (1) rudimentary otoscopic examination; (2) pure-tone screening; and, (3) immittance screening.

Visual Inspection

It will be useful here to discuss visual inspection of the ear. The possibility of appreciable hearing loss can usually be detected either by visual inspection by an otolaryngologist or by audiological testing. Heretofore, most audiologists have not been trained, even minimally, in otoscopic examination of the ear, presumably because of concern and respect for professional boundaries between the audiological and the medical professions. These boundaries must continue to be observed and respected. It seems a paradox, however, that audiology training programs spend considerable time in teaching students anatomy and physiology of the ear, but seem to actively discourage students from looking into a human external ear. Particularly after exposure to the auditory system through appropriate coursework, the student does not require a great deal of additional training in order to visualize congenital atresia, a foreign body or significant accumulation of cerumen in the ear canal, a reddened and inflamed ear canal or eardrum , or draining discharge. Certainly it is not within the audiologist's responsibilities to make a medical diagnosis on the basis of superficial otoscopic inspection of the ear, or even on the basis of detailed audiological tests. The responsibility for medical diagnosis belongs to the medical profession. On the other hand, any audiologist of average intelligence should be able to identify ear problems which would be obvious to any lay person.

The reluctance of audiologists to look inside the ear seems to be changing gradually due to the relatively recent addition of several test protocols to the audiologist's armamentarium. In recent years, audiologists have been actively engaged in immittance testing, in electronystagmographic testing, and in making earmold impressions for hearing aids. It is *necessary* for the audiologist to *look* inside the ear canal before inserting an immittance probe tip, directing a stream of water into an ear canal, or inserting a cotton wad followed by earmold impression material. The presumption is, of course, that obvious problems of the ear canal and tympanic membrane will be visualized.

On the basis of lack of training in otoscopy, it should be apparent that an audiologist will miss many ear problems which would be abundantly apparent to an otolaryngologist or other physician. On the other hand, physicians do not typically accomplish hearing screening in the schools. The point is that audiologists accomplishing hearing screening in the schools will miss even the visually obvious ear disorders if they fail to look. A second point is that there are other audiological tools to help identify possible hearing problems missed by the audiologist during rudimentary otoscopic inspection. The goal of elementary otoscopic examination of the ear canal accomplished by an audiologist is simply to identify obvious ear problems before other tests involved in the hearing screening battery are accomplished. Specifically, the audiologist should look for blockage of the ear canal, obvious inflammatory processes, and ear discharge. The visualization of any of these factors should, of course, lead to an immediate medical referral.

Pure-Tone Screening

A second source of significant information in the hearing screening battery is data from routine pure-tone sweep frequency screening tests of the type which have been conducted in the public schools for many years. In fact, pure-tone screening data have been, and, unfortunately, continue to be, the sole source of information relative to hearing loss in many school districts. Although there have been variations and refinements across the years, as indicated in Table 4-1, (Anderson, 1978; ASHA, 1975; Darley, 1961; Illinois: Department of Public Health, 1974; Northern and Downs, 1978), the typical pure tone hearing screening protocol involves monaural presentation of pure

Table 4-1.
Comparison of recommended test frequencies, intensity levels,
and pass/fail criteria for school hearing screening

Source of Data	Test Frequencies in KHz	Intensity Level in dB HL (ANSI—1969)	Pass/Fail Criteria
Nat. Conf. on I.D. Audiometry (Darley, 1961)	1K, 2K, 4K & 6K & 6KHz	20 dB @ 1K, 2K, & 6KHz. 30 dB @ 4KHz	Failure to hear tones in either ear.
Illinois Dept. of Public Health (1974)	.5K, 1K, 2K & 4KHz	25 or 35 dB	Failure to hear 1 tone at 35 dB in either ear, or 2 tones in 1 ear.
ASHA Comm. on Audiometric evaluation (1975)	1K, 2K, & 4KHz	20 dB @ 1KHz & 2KHz & 25 dB @ 4KHz	Failure to hear any frequency in either ear.
Northern & Downs (1978)	1K, 2K, 3K &/or 4K, and 6KHz	25 dB	Failure to hear 1 tone @ 1K or 2K, or 2 of 3 tones at 3K, 4K, or 6KHz.
Anderson (1978)	1K, 2K, & 4KHz	20 dB	Failure to hear any tone in either ear.
Downs (1968)	1K, 2K, 4K, & 6K or 8KHz	15 dB	Failure to hear either 1K or 2K, or both 4K and 6K/8K in either ear.

From Roeser R J and Downs M D *Auditory Disorders in School Children.* New York: Thieme-Stratton, Inc., 1981, p. 136. With permission.

tones between 500 and 4000 or 6000 Hz at an intensity of 20 or 25 dB HL to each ear.

The criterion for failure is usually failure to respond at any screening frequency in either ear. One reason for the selection of 20 or 25 dB HL as the screening level and as the criterion for failure is the assumption that children with hearing better than 20 or 25 dB HL do not have "educationally significant" hearing loss. Two major problems exist with the use of pure-tone sweep frequency screening in isolation. First, approximately 52 percent of children with active middle ear disease, who are in need of immediate medical attention, present pure-tone thresholds which are better than the 20 or 25 dB screening level and, consequently, are not identified. The second problem relates to the definition of "educationally significant" hearing loss. Some educators argue that, while it is the responsibility of the schools to identify educationally significant hearing loss, it is not the responsibility of the schools to identify medically significant hearing loss. Recent retrospective studies suggest that, even though thresholds may be better than 20 or 25 dB, children with middle ear disease have, in fact, educationally significant hearing loss (Blair, Peterson, & Viehweg, 1985; Quigley, 1970; Dobie & Berlin, 1979; Zinkus, Gottlieb, & Shapiro, 1978; Kessler & Randolph, 1979; Needleman, 1977). The magnitude of hearing loss in children with middle ear disease often fluctuates over time, so that hearing is substantially poorer during some periods than during others. Even in cases where the hearing loss does not fluctuate, children with 10–15 dB HL thresholds do not have "normal" hearing. Children with slight hearing loss (less than 25 dB HL) resulting from middle ear disease have been reported to experience progressive academic and speech/language delay, presumably as a consequence of missing many of the subtleties of auditory-verbal communication over a prolonged period of time (Eisen, 1962; Hodgett, 1982; Kaplan, Fleshman, Bender, et al. 1973; Holme & Kunze, 1969; Hersher, 1978; Howie, 1980; Masters & March, 1978; Freeman & Parkins, 1979; Kodman, 1963; Hook, 1979). Furthermore, children with latent and unresolved middle ear infection often do not feel well and do not have the energy or attention needed for optimum performance in the classroom.

Immittance Screening

If it is agreed that, in order to meet the educational needs of schoolchildren, it is important to identify "educationally significant" and "medically significant" hearing loss, and if it is agreed that pure-tone sweep frequency hearing screening does not identify a significant proportion of medically significant hearing problems, then some other method must be used to identify the medically significant problems. Various parameters of immittance audiometry are presently used to successfully identify a major proportion of medically significant hearing losses not identified using pure-tone sweep frequency screening. The specific parameters of the immittance battery that have been incorporated into hearing screening programs include tympanometry, middle ear pressure, physical volume, static compliance, and acoustic reflex. Two possible impedance screening protocols include the so-called Nashville Symposium (Bess, 1980) guidelines and the American Speech-Language-Hearing Association Guidelines (ASHA, 1979).

Combined Screening

A legitimate question must be raised relative to the additional time required when basic otoscopic inspection and immittance testing are added to the usual pure-tone screening testing. Basic otoscopic inspection and immittance measures can both be completed very quickly, but both, of course, require an increase in time commitment over that required for pure-tone screening alone. A partial solution to the time dilemma involves abbreviating each component of the screening program so that each is used to contribute the information which it is uniquely suited to provide. For example, some writers suggest deleting certain of the pure-tone frequencies from the protocol when rudimentary otoscopy and immittance measures are included in the screening battery. The American Speech and Hearing Association (ASHA, 1984) has proposed guidelines for identification audiometry which involves both pure-tone screening and immittance screening. Roeser and Northern (1981) have also presented recommended guidelines for a combined pure-tone and immittance screening program.

Screening Frequency

Given that time for hearing screening in the schools is limited, and given that evaluative efforts should be maximally productive in identifying children with possible hearing loss, one must determine which students in the schools should be screened and how often. It is generally agreed that the greatest effort should be concentrated on groups of school-age children known to experience a relatively high incidence of hearing loss. It has been reported, for example, that approximately 85 percent of children detected as having hearing loss in the schools will be detected by the third grade (Corliss & Watson, 1961). Children in the primary grades seem to be prone to hearing loss associated with otitis media. Major emphasis should therefore be directed toward identifying children with hearing loss in the early grades. The typical procedure is to screen children annually in kindergarten and grades one, two, and three and to screen not less often than every third year thereafter. For example, the school system may elect to screen children in kindergarten and grades one, two, three, six, nine, and twelve.

In addition to the screening conducted during these scheduled grades, certain of the children should be screened at other times. For example, each child new to the district should be screened in order to obtain baseline data and data relative to adequacy of hearing. Pupils identified in previous screening programs as having auditory impairment should be monitored closely so that resolution or progression of hearing loss can be charted. Children with delayed or defective speech and language skills should receive hearing screening testing to rule out hearing loss as a possible etiological factor in the developmental delay. Children returning to school following a lengthy or serious illness should be screened to rule out the possibility that the illness resulted in loss of hearing. In addition, children in remedial and special education programs should be screened to rule out hearing loss as a factor contributing to the need for remedial and special educational services.

It is vital to screen children who are referred by parents and other educational personnel, especially teachers, who suspect the possibility of hearing loss. Parents and teachers spend considerable time with children and are in a unique position to be aware of symptoms often associated with hearing loss, such as frequent requests for repetition, consistent turning of the head to the side, an excessively loud or quiet voice, obvious strain in trying to hear, visual fixation on the face of the teacher or parent, inattention during classroom discussion, frequent mistakes in following directions, tendency toward isolation and passivity, tension and lack of energy, speech impairment, and an obvious gap between judged potential and academic performance.

The validity and reliability of audiometric results, whether screening or threshold data, are based on several requisites, including: (1) competence of the tester(s); (2) accuracy of the instrumentation utilized; (3) adequacy of the environment relative to competing noise levels; and, of course, (4) the cooperation of the child.

Personnel Training

It must be assumed that the personnel used to secure screening data are adequately trained and capable of obtaining valid and reliable screening results. If audiologists and/or speech-language pathologist are not directly used in obtaining screening results, it is usually recommended that non-professional technical assistants undertake at least one college-level course which includes both didactic information and hands-on-experience. The technical assistants utilized in screening must be closely supervised and the data carefully monitored by the educational audiologist.

Calibration

Calibration accuracy of the instrumentation used for screening must be carefully monitored during data acquisition. The likelihood is substantial that failure to monitor calibration accuracy will lead to invalid test results (Thomas, Preslar, Summers & Stewart, 1969). An electroacoustic calibration check should be performed prior to beginning hearing screening data acquisition and calibration discrepancies should be resolved. With a little planning, it is usually possible to secure on-site calibration services provided by a factory-trained and certified person if an audiometer is in need of such services. A sound-level meter with an associated 6 cc coupler should be used often during the data acquisition process to monitor intensity accuracy and a "biological check" of the instruments used should be performed at least daily by the person(s) using the equipment.

Table 4-2.
Approximate octave band levels allowable for screening at
20–25 dB level recommended by the ASHA Committee on
Audiometric evaluations (dB SPL)

Test frequency	500	1000	2000	4000
Octave band cutoff frequencies	300 600	600 1200	1200 2400	2400 4800
Allowable ambient noise for threshold at zero HL (re: ANSI-1969)	26	30	38	51
Plus ASHA screening level (re: ANSI-1969)	20	20	20	25
Resultant maximum ambient noise allowable for ASHA screening	46	50	58	76

Ambient Noise

Hearing screening data is of little value when obtained in an environment where children cannot hear at the screening criterion level(s) due to noise in the environment. In a noisy test environment, the audiologist cannot be certain whether lack of a response from a child is because of inability to hear due to hearing loss or inability to hear due to noise masking (Darley, 1961). Audiologists must frequently assess the possible effect of noise on screening data by assuring themselves that they can themselves hear the various pure tones at the criterion intensities. If a sound-level meter is available, decibel measurements can be made in the octave or one-third octave bands surrounding the various frequencies included in the screening regimen. Publications, including the American Speech and Hearing Association Committee on Audiometric Evaluation Guidelines for Identification Audiometry (ASHA, 1975) and the American National Standards Institute Criteria for Background Noise in Audiometer Rooms (1977), have listed allowable ambient noise levels for audiometric test environments. The ASHA values appear in Table 4-2. These publications have listed maximum allowable background decibel SPL levels in order to measure auditory thresholds to "zero" decibels HL using the ANSI 1969 norm (ANSI, 1970) at various frequencies. When accomplishing hearing screening rather than threshold testing, the audiologist can add the value of the screening level to the values indicated above.

A significant factor in the success of the identification program is the cooperation and commitment of school personnel and parents. Many techniques can be used to develop mutual understanding and cooperation. The educational audiologist can attend staff meetings and parent/teacher association meetings and explain the reasons for the program along with pertinent details about the testing. Teachers may resent having their classes interrupted and some parents may refuse to have their children's hearing tested unless they can see the potential benefit which may be derived for their students and children. The educational audiologist may find it helpful to present a brief historical review which summarizes results from hearing screenings conducted in previous years.

A published schedule of testing issued well in advance of such testing and the securing of permission slips from parents well in advance can also serve to minimize frustrations and perceived interruptions. Teachers can be extremely helpful in handling the logistics of getting children to and from the hearing screening area, maintaining order, supplying class lists, and filling out demographic data. When appropriate cooperative relationships are formed, the school nurse can also be helpful, particularly in helping parents to take care of recommended post-screening medical follow-up. A factor of prime importance in securing and maintaining the support of educational personnel is making certain they receive prompt information concerning the individual results of the tests and making certain that the appropriate data becomes a part of the child's educational file as quickly as possible. Examples of forms that may be used in tabulating data and communicating or transmiting information to interested people are shown by Anderson (1978). Personal interviews with teachers of children with hearing problems can do much to build mutual understanding and cooperation and can be vital in optimizing the learning situation for the hearing-impaired child. Suggestions and recommendations can be discussed and explained as appropriate during these interviews.

Ordinarily, children who fail the initial hearing screening test are rescreened after a period of approximately 2 weeks. The second screening is conducted to confirm the presence of possible hearing loss identified in the initial screening and to identify those children who may have misunderstood instructions or failed to cooperate appropriately for some other reason. The second screening is also conducted to clear those children who may have had a transient hearing loss on the date of the initial screening test.

AUDIOLOGICAL EVALUATION

General Considerations

Once a child has failed the second screening test, the identification phase of the program is completed. The task now becomes one of detailing the parameters of the hearing loss and initiating (re)habilitation measures. As a first step, and at the very least, the educational audiologist should schedule all children who fail the second screening test for pure-tone threshold testing.

It is to be hoped that the educational audiologist possesses the requisite clinical skills to perform a full basic comprehensive audiological evaluation.

Some school districts do not have instrumentation available to accomplish audiological testing beyond pure-tone screening and pure-tone air-conduction threshold testing. Other distrcts are equipped to provide a range of basic audiological services, including pure-tone air- and bone-conduction testing, speech audiometric measures including SRT, speech discrimination in quiet and noise, most comfortable and uncomfortable listening levels, an immittance battery, central auditory abilities testing, and some special auditory tests. If audiological services can be provided within the school system, the available testing should be completed before referring the child to an outside audiologist or physician. If the recommended audiological testing cannot be provided in the schools, the child should be referred to an outside audiologist for audiological testing. Care must be exercised to fully inform parents concerning the need for audiological data and the educational audiologist must obtain the necessary release of information forms before a report can be sent to an outside referral source.

Following audiological evaluation, wherein the specific parameters of the hearing loss are detailed, the child should be referred to a physician (preferably an otolaryngologist) for any possible medical and/or surgical treatment. If a family practitioner or pediatrician serves as the medical manager for the children of the family involved, care must be exercised to make sure this physician is included in the process. A full audiological report should reach the physician *before* the child is seen for medical examination. Steps must also be taken to ensure that a report be received *from* the physician concerning medical/surgical treatment and recommendations. In many cases, it will be necessary to send a written request for such a report to the physician. The return rate will likely be greatest if a prepared form is provided for the physician to fill out and return to the educational audiologist. Steps must also be initiated to assure that any medical/surgical recommedations are carried out. When children are identified who have hearing loss of sufficient magnitude to be of educational significance, but for whom medical and/or surgical intervention is not indicated, the educational audiologist must initiate action to obtain a wearable amplification system (see Chapter 5) and must also initiate other aural (re)habilitation programs to optimize the child's educational experience.

It is not the purpose of the present chapter to present information related to specific audiological test protocols. Several excellent sources exist which deal with the specific methodology to be used in pure-tone air- and bone-conduction threshold testing. The reader is referred to a classic article by Carhart and Jerger (1959) entitled "Preferred Method for Clinical Determination of Pure-Tone Thresholds." Excellent chapters exist in several textbooks which cover audiometric technique in air- and bone-conduction testing with masking and speech audiometry (Green, in Katz, 1978; Wilber, in Rintelmann,

1979; Hodgson, 1980; Wilson & Margolis and Bess, in Konkle & Rintelmann, 1983).

Younger school-age children with hearing loss and children with special problems often present reduced responsiveness and inability to attend fully. In testing these children, it will often be necessary for the audiologist to vary the testing paradigm from that used with older children and adults. There are, of course, audiometric techniques and materials that have been developed specifically for use with young children. For example, when accomplishing pure-tone testing, it may be necessary to resort to "conditioned play audiometry" in order to maintain interest in the auditory task at hand. In other cases, it may be necessary to add the use of "tangible reinforcers" such as M&M's, sugared cereal, raisins, trinkets, etc. in order to develop sufficient motivation and attention. Audiologists must arm themselves with a number of different "fun" activities and tangible reinforcers so as to appeal to a broad range of children. All children will not enjoy throwing blocks in a box and all children will not work for "Fruit Loops." The specific techniques used in obtaining audiological data for school-age children are limited only by the imagination and creativity of the audiologists. It is much easier for audiologists to feel comfortable in varying audiological technique when they operate from a solid theoretical/information base, thoroughly understand the instrumentation to be used, have a broad range of clinical materials and supplies, and have sufficient experience to relate effectively on an interpersonal basis with children.

The audiologist working with school-age children must continually ask the questions: "What types of information do I need from this child?" "What can I do clinically to demonstrate, describe, and quantify the auditory difficulties this child seems to present on a daily basis?" "What tools and techniques can I use to get the information given the set of circumstances with which I am *now* faced?" The direction of the audiological evaluation and decisions concerning the specific tests to be included in the battery must often be revised based on data received during the evaluation. For example, a child may be referred by a classroom teacher with an observation that the child finds it difficult to attend in class and frequently cannot follow sequential directions. The difficulty may be related to any one or a combination of several factors and the audiologist must systematically rule out potential causative factors. The audiologist may find normal sensitivity for pure tones and for speech and normal acuity for speech when presented in quiet. At this juncture, the audiologist should recognize that the difficulties are very likely not related to peripheral hearing loss and other avenues must be explored. In this situation, the audiologist may want to obtain such data as speech discrimination scores in noise or obtain data from behavioral tests used in the "central auditory abilities" battery.

It must be remembered when working with young children that the attention span and length of time over which valid and reliable data can be obtained may be limited. The educational audiologist must obtain the most critical and useful information early in the evaluation and leave the frills for later. For example, the educational audiologist may wish to obtain speech audiometric data first, since this information may, in some respects, relate more directly than other data to educational progress and be easier for nonaudiological educational personnel to understand. In accomplishing pure-tone testing, the educational audiologist may initially want to obtain only a low-, middle-, and high-frequency pure-tone air-conduction threshold from each ear and a low- and high-frequency unmasked bone-conduction threshold. In fact, the audiologist may wish to bypass bone conduction testing with masking if tympanometric findings are normal. If the child is still attending when the most important information is secured, then the audiologist may wish to go back and fill in the gaps.

Pure-Tone Audiometry

Humans are not ordinarily exposed to pure tones as common environmental stimuli and, for this reason, pure tones have relatively low face validity as a stimulus with which to measure functional auditory skills. Nevertheless, while not directly related to day-to-day function, pure-tone thresholds provide important diagnostic and prognostic information concerning degree of hearing loss across the frequency spectrum utilized for speech reception. The various phonemes of speech are significantly different in terms of their spectral characteristics, and the nature of the pure-tone audiometric configuration will have important implications for the educational audiologist relative to speech and language programming, selection of appropriate electroacoustic amplification parameters, and need for medical and other special services.

Magnitude of hearing loss has been defined on the basis of the pure-tone average of the speech frequencies (500, 1000, and 2000 Hz). A rather common descriptive categorization of hearing loss involves the amount of hearing lost: normal range, 0–15 db; slight hearing loss range, 16–25 dB; mild hearing loss range, 26–40 dB; moderate hearing loss range, 41–55 dB; moderately severe hearing loss range, 56–70 dB; severe hearing loss range, 71–90 dB, profound hearing loss, over 91 dB. While such a categorization has some descriptive utility, many other factors contribute significantly to the handicapping nature of the hearing loss, or to the ability of the child to compensate for the loss in hearing sensitivity. Some of these secondary factors include age at onset, etiology of the hearing loss, speech discriminatory capacity, intelligence, motivation, excellence of training, presence of other handicapping conditions, and familial support and cooperation.

Immittance Audiometry

As mentioned earlier, middle ear disease constitutes a major cause of hearing loss in the schools, particulary in the earlier grades. The tool which is of most use to the audioloigist in detecting the presence of middle ear disease and in monitoring progression of and resolution of middle ear disease is the immittance bridge/meter. Tympanometry is a powerful tool for detecting the presence of middle ear effusion and the measurement of middle ear pressure is useful in detecting eustachian tube malfunction. The physical volume measurement is helpful in detecting the presence of an open tympanic membrane perforation or in assessing the patency of pressure equalization tubes, and ipsilateral and contralateral acoustic reflex measurements provide important information concerning both conductive and sensorineural hearing loss. In a recent survey (Martin & Sides, 1985), 93 percent of audiologists were found to use immittance testing routinely in their practice.

Speech Audiometry

Speech audiometry is a highly useful tool in obtaining information concerning speech sensitivity and acuity in various situations. The speech reception threshold provides a measure of degree or magnitude of hearing loss for speech and should agree closely with the pure-tone average of the speech frequencies (500, 1000, and 2000 Hz). Picture representations of spondee words or tangible toy representations of spondee words can be used when children are unable to repeat these words in the usual way.

One closed-set response test which has been developed for measuring the threshold for speech is included in the Threshold by Picture Identification test (TIP) (Siegenthaler & Haspiel, 1966; Siegenthaler, 1975). The audiologist may need to depart from using standard spondee word materials in measuring thresholds for speech and ask the child questions regarding things which are within that child's response vocabulary or which are of sufficient interest to stimulate responsiveness.

Speech discrimination scores provide suprathreshold information relative to capacity of the child to differentiate among and betewen the various phonemes of speech. The familiar CID W-22 test lists (Hirsh, Davis, Silverman, Reynolds, Eldert, & Bensen, 1952) and the NU6 test lists (Tillman & Carhart, 1966) are among the various speech test lists that can be used successfully for older children; several speech discrimination test lists have been developed specifically for use with younger children. These tests include the phonetically balanced familiar word lists—PBF (Hudgins, 1944), the phonetically balanced kindergarten word lists—PBK (Haskins, 1949), Word Intelligibility by Picture Identification—WIPI (Ross & Lerman, 1970), the Discrimination by Identification of Pictures—DIP (Siegenthaler & Haspiel, 1966), the Northwestern

University Children's Perception of Speech Test—NU-CHIPS (Katz & Elliot, 1978), the Pediatric Speech Intelligibility test—PSI (Jerger, Lewis, Hawkins, and Jerger, 1980), the Sound Effects Recognition Test—SERT (Finitzo-Hieber, Gerlin, Matkin, & Cherow-Skalka, 1980), the California Consonant Test (Owens & Shubert, 1977), and the Auditory Numbers Test—ANT (Erber, 1980).

In addition to the single-sound or word-discrimination materials in common use, sentence tests have also been developed which are supposed to provide higher face validity and a more realistic approach to simulation of speech materials encountered in everyday communication. Sentence tests that have been developed include the WIPI sentences (Weber & Reddel, 1976), Synthetic Sentence Identification tests—SSI and SSIC (Jerger, 1970; Wilson, 1978), the Blair Sentences (Blair, 1976), the Speech Perception in Noise—SPIN (Kalikow, Stevens & Elliot, 1977; Elliot, 1979), and the sentence portion of the PSI (Jerger et al., 1980).

Some of the above materials are open-set response tests and others utilize a closed-set response format. Some of the materials are suitable for very young children and others are useful only for older children and adults. Some of the materials utilize single-word presentation and single-word response and some of the materials utilize multiple-word presentation and response. Some of the materials involve significant contextual cueing while others provide little or no contextual cueing. Some of the tests involve presentation of speech against a background of noise while others do not. Scoring procedures vary among the various tests and interpretation of results must be considered in relation to the normative data available. From the writers' perspective, there is no "best" speech audiometric test. The audiologist must be familiar with the materials available and must be sufficiently flexible to use these and/or other techniques to provide the information needed for a particular child. The speech audiometric materials available with which to measure speech recognition for school-age children has vastly expanded over the past 15 years. Any of the test materials can be presented against a background of noise of one type or another. It is helpful to obtain data concerning a particular child's responses to speech under optimal listening conditions, but it also seems important to obtain information in situations which, to some extent, approximate the noisy conditions encountered in many classrooms. Again, various types of background or "noise" have been used in measuring speech reception in the presence of competition. The competition sources have included white noise, speech spectrum noise, sentence material from a single talker, meaningful connected discourse from a single talker, and meaningful connected discourse from multiple talkers. Research is needed to provide information concerning the disruptive effects of various competition sources on the scores obtained while using the different speech materials and data is needed concerning differences related to the age ranges of school age children.

The primary goal of the audiological evaluation in the school setting is to obtain data that can be used to explain educational difficulties and data which can be used in developing educational and aural (re)habilitation strategies. This is not meant to leave the impression that data relative to the medical aspects of the hearing loss are not important. Data related to the etiology and site of lesion in the auditory system are critical to the overall decision-making processes. The primary business of the schools is, however, education and the physician will likely not be primarily interested in securing data related to educational factors. The educational audiologist *must* obtain educationally relevant audiological data.

Special Auditory Tests

The educational audiologist working in the schools may or may not have the instrumentation capacity to allow audiological testing beyond the basic comprehensive audiological evaluation and immittance battery. In this case, the educational audiologist must refer to an outside audiologist who specializes in the type of testing needed. For example, once a child with apparent auditory difficulties has been shown not to have a peripheral hearing loss, the educational audiologist may find it necessary to refer the child to an audiologist who specializes in central auditory abilities testing, to a learning disabilities specialist for evaluation of possible attention deficit disorder, or to a psychologist for a psycho-social evaluation (see Chapter 3). In another instance, a child may be found with a progressive sensori-neural hearing loss. In this case, the educational audiologist may wish to refer the child concurrently to an otolaryngologist for medical evaluation and to an audiologist who specializes in site-of-lesion testing. Medical evaluation and site-of-lesion testing are important in both bilateral and unilateral progressive sensori-neural hearing loss, but are particularly important in the presence of unilateral progressive sensori-neural hearing loss so that a determination can be made relative to what pathological processes affect one ear but not the other.

Traditional site-of-lesion testing is often difficult to accomplish with young children due to the exacting nature of the tasks involved and the absolute requirement for total concentration on the part of the child. Special applications of acoustic reflex testing and auditory brainstem-evoked response testing (ABR) may be indicated in these cases for 2 reasons. First, acoustic reflex measurements and brainstem-evoked response evaluation do not require active cooperation on the part of the child. In fact, children must often be sedated in order to obtain ABR test results. Second, auditory brain-stem-evoked response is a very powerful tool in detecting retrocochlear auditory pathology. The indiciators of ABR abnormality include prolonged interpeak latencies, abnormal Wave I versus Wave V amplitude ratios, and abnormal latency shifts and wave form degeneration resulting from increasing the click rate. The ABR evaluation is highly sensitive to problems along the VIII nerve or in the auditory tracts of the brain stem, but is not specific to the disease process. Abnormal ABR findings do not indicate the presence of a space-occupying lesion, but do indicate that there is, or has been, an insult to the auditory tracts of the VIII nerve or the brainstem. When abnormal ABR responses are found, however, the possibility definitely exists that a space-occupying lesion is present.

Although relatively rare in children, space-occupying lesions can be very serious and the earlier they are detected and removed, the better. It is important to realize that abnormal brainstem-evoked response findings can occur as a result of brain damage and can result in learning disorders. There are several reports of children with learning disorders who demonstrate normal hearing as measured using an audiometer, and who have no observable or detectable auditory lesion, but who have grossly abnormal brainstem-evoked response findings. The number of children with learning disorders who evidence abnormal ABR findings are in a significant minority, however, and, at the moment, ABR testing does not seem to be an economical way to detect learning disorders, either from the standpoint of "yield" or sensitivity or from the standpoint of monetary investment. Furthermore, ABR testing is certainly not the best way of obtaining threshold information from school-age children who are capable of responding reliably to routine test techniques. On the other hand, ABR is a very useful tool in detecting the presence of possible hearing loss in the high-frequency region above 1500 Hz in difficult-to-test children who cannot respond appropriately in behavioral testing. Middle latency-evoked response measures have been used with some success in measurement of hearing in the lower frequencies.

REFERENCES

American national standard specifications for audiometers (ANSI S3.6-1969). New York: American National Standards Institute, Inc. 1970.

American National Standards Institute. American standard criteria for background noise in audiometer rooms (ANSI S3.1-1977). New York: American National Standards Institute, Inc., 1977.

American Speech and Hearing Association (ASHA), Committee on Audiometric Evaluation. Guidelines for identification audiometry. *ASHA*, 1975, *17*, 94–99.

American Speech and Hearing Association (ASHA), Committee on Audiometric Evaluation. Guidelines for acoustic immittance function. *ASHA*, 1979, *21*, 283–288.

American Speech-Language-Hearing Association (ASLHA). Proposed revisions of guidelines for identification audiometry. *ASHA,* 1984, *26,* 47–50.

Anderson C C. Hearing screening for children. In J Katz (Ed.), *Handbook of clinical audiology* (ed. 2). Baltimore: Williams and Wilkins, 1978. pp. 48-60.

Bess F H. Impedance screening for children: A need for more research. *Annals Otology Rhinology Laryngology,* 1980, Suppl. 68, 228–232

Blair J C. The contributing influences of amplification, speechreading, and classroom environments on the ability of hard of hearing children to discriminate sentences. Unpublished doctoral dissertation, Northwestern University, 1976.

Blair J C. Peterson, M E, & Viehweg, S H. The effect of mild sensorineural hearing loss on academic performance among school age children. *The Volta Review,* 1985, Vol 87, 87–94.

Carhart R & Jerger J. Preferred method for clinical determination of pure-tone thresholds. *Journal of Speech and Hearing Disorders,* 1959, *24,* 330–345.

Corliss L & Watson J. A school system studies the effectiveness of routine audiometry. *Journal of Health, Physical Education and Recreation of the National Educational Association,* March, 1961, p. 27.

Darley F L. Identification audiometry for school-age children: Basic procedures. *Journal of Speech and Hearing Disorders,* 1961, Monograph Suppl. 9, pp. 26-34.

Dobie R A & Berlin C I. Influence of otitis media on hearing and development, *Annals of Otology, Rhinology, and Laryngology* 1979, *88,* (Suppl. 60). 48–53.

Downs M P. Auditory screening. *The Otolaryngologic Clinics of North America* 1968, *11,* 611–629.

Eagles E L, Wishik S M, Doerfler L G, Melnick W, & Levine H S. Hearing sensitivity and related factors in children. *Laryngoscope,* June 1963.

Eisen N H. Some effects of early sensory deprivation on later behavior: The quondam hard-of-hearing child. *Journal of Abnormal Social Psychology,* 1962, *65,* 338.

Elliott L L. Performance of children aged 9 to 17 years on a test of speech intelligibility in noise using sentence material with controlled predictability. *Journal of the Acoustical Society of America,* 1979, *66,* 651–662.

Erber N P. Use of the auditory numbers test to evaluate speech perception abilities of hearing-impaired children. *Journal of Speech and Hearing Disorders,* 1980, *45,* 527–532.

Finitzo-Hieber T. Gerlin I J, Matkin N D, & Cherow-Skalka E. A sound effects recognition test for the pediatric evaluation. *Ear and Hearing,* 1980, *1,* 271–276.

Freeman B A & Parkins C. The prevalence of middle ear disease among learning disabled children. *Clinical Pediatrics,* 1979, *18,* 205–212.

Haskins H A. A phonetically balanced test of speech discrimination for children. Unpublished master's thesis, Northwestern University, 1949.

Hersher L. Minimal brain dysfunction and otitis media. *Perceptual and Motor Skills,* 1978, *47,* 723–726.

Hirsh I J, Davis H, Silverman S R, Reynolds E G, Eldert E, & Bensen R W. Development of materials for speech audiometry. *Journal of Speech and Hearing Disorders,* 1952, *17,* 321–337.

Hodgett J. Chronic otitis media and language delay in a select population. Unpublished master's thesis. Utah State University, 1982.

Hodgson W R. *Basic audiologic evaluation.* Baltimore: Williams and Wilkins, 1980.

Holme V A & Kunze L H. Effects of chronic otitis media on language and speech development. *Pediatrics* 1969, *43,* 833–838.

Hook P E. Learning disabilities in the hearing impaired, *Ear, Nose and Throat Journal,* 1979, *58,* 40–52.

Howie V M. Developmental sequelae of chronic otitis media, a review. *Develop. Behav. Pediatr.* March 1980. pp. 34–38.

Hudgins C V. A method of appraising the speech of the deaf, *Volta Review,* 1944, *51,* 597–601.

Illinois Department of Public Health. *A manual for audiometrists.* Springfield, Ill., 1974.

Jerger J. Development of synthetic sentence identification (SSI) as a tool for speech audiometry. In C Rojskjer (Ed.). *Speech audiometry.* Second Danavox Symposium, Andelsbogtrykkeriet i Odense, Denmark, 1970, 44–650.

Jerger S, Lewis S, Hawkins J, & Jerger J. Pediatric Speech Intelligibility Test. I. Generation of test materials. *International Journal Pediatric Otorhinolaryngology,* 1980, *2,* 217–230.

Kalikow D N, Stevens K N, & Elliot L L. Development of a test of speech intelligibility in noise using sentence materials with controlled word predictability. *Journal of the Acoustical Society of America,* 1977, *61,* 1337–1351.

Kaplan G K, Fleshman J K, Bender T R, Baum, C, & Clark P S. Long term effects of otitis media: A ten year cohort study of Alaska Eskimo children. *Pediatrics,* 1973, *52,* 577–585.

Katz J. (Ed.). *Handbook of clinical audiology* (ed. 2).Baltimore: Williams and Wilkins, 1978.

Katz J & Elliot L L. Development of a new children's speech discrimination test. Paper presented at the National Convention of the American Speech-Language-Hearing Association, Chicago, November, 1978.

Kessler M E & Randolph K. The effects of early middle ear disease on the auditory abilities of third grade children. *Journal of the Academy of Rehabilitative Audiology,* 1979, *12,* 6–20.

Kodman F. Educational status of hard-of-hearing children in the classroom. *Journal of Speech and Hearing Research* 1963, *28,* 297–299.

Konkle D F & Rintelmann W F. (eds.). *Principles of speech audiometry.* Baltimore; University Park Press, 1983.

Martin F N & Sides D G. Survey of Current Audiometric practices. *ASHA,* 1985, *27,* 29–36.

Masters L & March G E. Middle ear pathology as a factor in learning disabilities. *Journal of Learning Disabilities,* 1978, *2,* 54–57.

Needleman H. Effects of hearing loss from early recurrent otitis media on speech and language development. In B Jaffe, (ed.), *Hearing loss in children.* Baltimore; University Park Press, 1977.

Northern J L & Downs M P. Identification audiometry with children. In J L Northern & M P Downs (ed.), *Hearing in children* (ed. 2). Baltimore : Williams and Wilkins, 1978. pp. 193–224.

Owens E & Shubert E D. Development of the California Consonant Test. *Journal of Speech and Hearing Research,* 1977, *20,* 463–474.

Quigley S P. Some effects of hearing impairment upon school performance. Prepared for the Division of Special Education Services, Office of the Superintendent of Public Instruction, State of Illinois, 1970.

Rintelmann W F (Ed.). *Hearing assesment.* Baltimore: University Park Press, 1979.

Roeser R J & Downs M D. *Auditory Disorders in School Children.* New York: Thieme-Stratton, Inc. 1981, p. 136.

Roeser R J & Northern J L. Screening for hearing loss and middle ear disorders. In R J Roeser & M P Downs (Eds.), *Auditory disorders in school children.* Thieme-Stratton, New York: 1981.

Ross M. & Lerman J. A picture identification test for hearing impaired children. *Journal of Speech and Hearing Research,* 1970, *5,* 44–72.

Siegenthaler B. Reliability of the TIP and DIP speech-hearing tests for children. *Journal of Communication Disorders,* 1975, *8,* 325–333.

Siegenthaler B & Haspeil G. Development of two standardized measures of hearing for speech by children. U. S. Department of Health, Education, and Welfare, Project No 2372, Contract No. OE-5-10-003, 1966.

Thomas W, Preslar M, Summers R, & Stewart J. Calibration and working condition of 100 audiometers. Washington, D. C.; *Public Health Report,* 1969, *84,* 311–327.

Tillman T W & Carhart R. An expanded test for speech discrimination utilizing CNC monosyllabic words. (Northwestern University Auditory Test No. 6, Technical Report No. SAM-TR-66-55). Brooks Air Force Base, Texas: USAF School of Aerospace Medicine, 1966.

Weber S & Redell R C. A sentence test of measuring speech discrmination in children. *Audiology and Hearing Education,* 1976, *2,* 30; 40.

Wilson M D Development and analysis of a simplified synthetic sentence identification test. Unpublished doctoral dissertation, Vanderbilt University, 1978.

Zinkus P W, Gottlieb M L, & Shapiro M. Developmental and psychoeducational sequelae of chronic otitis media. *American Journal of Disabled Children* 1978, *132,* 1100–1104.

Steven H. Viehweg

5
Hearing Aids

Hearing loss, of whatever cause, can and often does result in reduction or delay in communicative efficiency, educational progress, speech and language development, and social/emotional adjustment (see Chapter 4). Many children in the schools who evidence hearing loss suffer from mild and transient conductive hearing loss of short duration. Medical and/or surgical intervention often is successful in restoring hearing in these children. Some conductive hearing loss, however, is recurrent and less amenable to permanent resolution by medical or surgical treatment. In spite of the fact that the loss in these children is potentially resolvable, the children suffer the educational/communicational/social consequences of reduced hearing during active periods of the middle ear disease. Other children suffer from sensori-neural auditory pathology in which the resulting hearing loss is permanent and irreversible and not amenable to medical treatment.

A major and obvious result of either conductive or sensori-neural hearing loss is that the children affected do not hear well. Given that any indicated medical/surgical treatment has been completed, and given that hearing loss is still present, there is only one answer to the major problem (namely, that *the child does not hear well*). Amplification is the only remaining avenue to improve hearing. Such a statement is not meant to demean the many and significant benefits that can and do occur through other interventive strategies such as speechreading, auditory training, language/speech therapy, vocabulary development, special tutoring, and so on. The fact remains, however, that such treatments neither increase the physical intensity of sound nor improve auditory thresholds. Only use of amplification will result in such changes and, indeed, the provision of appropriate and optimal amplification may reduce the necessity or need for therapeutic intervention and/or improve the results of aural (re)habilitation when it is still necessary. For these reasons, many audiologists agree that use of amplification systems should be seriously considered for children with hearing loss of appreciable duration. This chapter will be devoted to a discussion of principles involved in choosing an appropriate amplification system and in managing the hearing aid(s) after completion of the fitting.

HEARING AID STYLES

Body Hearing Aids

Hearing aids may be obtained in four basic configurations: (1) body worn; (2) eyeglasses; (3) behind-the-ear; and, (4) in-the-ear/canal (see Fig. 5-1). Although body aids are still used in special circumstances, these instruments seem to have largely passed from the scene of amplification systems (Cranmer, 1984; Mahon, 1984; Skafte, 1984). Body aids are relatively bulky and heavy. Directional cues are reduced to some extent due to the location of the microphone on the body, and friction noise from clothing and other items poses a signal-to-noise problem. Furthermore, the location of the hearing aid against the body creates a baffle effect which, in essence, reduces or prevents amplification in the higher frequencies. There seems to be a significant consmetic/vanity factor to discourage the use of body hearing aids among older school-age children. With improvements in design and quality of hearing aid circuitry and with significant reduction in component size, hearing aid manufacturers have been able to package very powerful hearing aids in eyeglasses temple pieces or in cases worn behind the ear. On occasion, it is still not possible to obtain needed power from an ear-level instrument without acoustic feedback. In these instances, it may be necessary to use a body aid which increases the distance between the transducers of the hearing aid (microphone and receiver) and allows greater amplification without feedback.

Eyeglasses Hearing Aids

Eyeglasses hearing aids constitute one style of ear-level hearing aid system. The circuit components of the hearing aid are contained within the temple piece(s) of a pair of eyeglasses. Whereas a body hearing aid utilizes an external receiver, eyeglasses and other ear-level instruments utilize internal hearing aid receivers, i.e., receivers which are inside the chassis or case of the hearing aid itself. Eyeglasses hearing aids were quite popular among adult hearing aid users for several years when ear-level hearing aids were relatively larger than is the case at present. Since it has been possible to reduce the

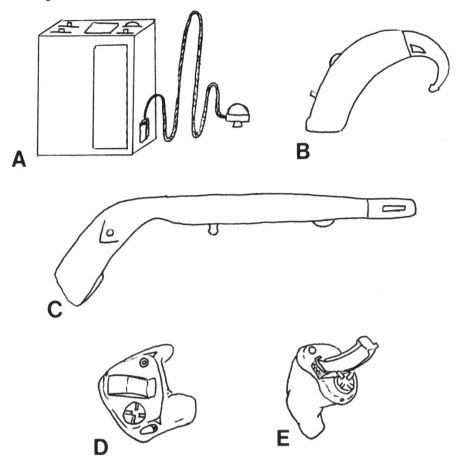

Fig. 5-1. Hearing aid types: (A) body aid, (B) behind-the-ear, (C) eyeglasses, (D) in-the-ear, and (E) in-the-canal.

size of behind-the-ear hearing aids substantially, however, use of eyeglasses hearing aids has been reduced.

There are several inherent disadvantages to eyeglasses hearing aids, particularly for use with children. For example, most eyeglasses hearing aids have been designed to fit an adult head and different lengths of extension tips have been used to adjust to individual differences. Even with the shortest possible extension tip, many eyeglasses hearing aids will not fit young children. Furthermore, eyeglasses instruments are more difficult than other aids to fit and adjust initially. After the initial fitting, active children are prone to bump or otherwise abuse eyeglasses hearing aids fairly often so that maintaining proper alignment and adjustment over a prolonged period of time is difficult. It is very difficult to provide "loaner" eyeglasses hearing aids and the inconvenience when use of a hearing aid or a pair of eyeglasses is lost is compounded when the user must be without both the hearing aid *and* the eyeglasses when one or the other is being repaired. For these and other reasons, eyeglasses hearing aid systems are not particularly practical for use with school-age children.

Post-Auricle Hearing Aids

Post-auricle or behind-the-ear hearing aids seem to be the amplification system of choice for school-age children for several practical reasons. First, data concerning the exact nature of the hearing loss may be somewhat sketchy and incomplete, particularly for younger school-age children with problems in addition to hearing loss. The multivariable controls on post-auricle hearing aids make it possible to change electroacoustic characteristics of the hearing aid system as specifications are revised based on increased information. Second, particularly in the case of mild conductive hearing loss, the gain and output of the hearing aid may need to be changed from time to time based on the fluctuation of the hearing loss. Third, it is possible to use loaner behind-the-ear instruments in order to assure consistent and continuous amplification when it is necessary to send a child's own hearing aid system in for factory repairs. This is difficult to accomplish with in-the-ear hearing aids. Fourth, as the size of the ear canal changes, earmolds often need to be changed in growing children. It is much less expensive to change an earmold than to change an entire hearing aid system as would be necessary for a custom in-the-ear hearing aid.

In-The-Ear/Canal Hearing Aids

In-the-ear hearing aids seem to be less appropriate for children than post-auricle hearing aids for the reasons explained above. Briefly, loaner in-the-ear hearing aids are difficult to provide when a hearing aid must be repaired. While some in-the-ear hearing aids have variable controls, there is not sufficient room in the in-the-ear shell (particularly in the case of children's smaller ears) for as many controls as is possible in other aids, and the ones included seem to provide a narrower range of variability than is the case with behind-the-ear instruments. While it is possible to use build-up-material on the shell of an in-the-ear hearing aid to reduce feedback when the aid becomes loose due to growth of the child, such a solution is often less effective than the provision of a new shell or earmold.

While in-the-ear hearing aids are worn with great success by many adult listeners (who are usually very careful with their instruments), use of in-the-ear hearing aids with children should be viewed with some skepticism. The authors can see no application of in-the-canal instruments for young children at the present time. The danger of loss, the difficulty of manipulating the controls, and problems associated with maintaining an appropriate seal in the ear canal seem to contraindicate use of in-the-canal instruments with young children.

Use of in-the-ear hearing aids may have some applicability for responsible teenaged students who have attained a major portion of growth and who have hearing loss in a magnitude range which can be reached successfully with an in-the-ear hearing aid. Teenaged students can be extremely sensitive concerning cosmetic appearance and will do almost anything at times to reduce the sense of being different. The adage which states that "the best hearing aid in the world is the one the client will wear" may literally be true in the case of teenaged school students. They may simply refuse to wear anything but an in-the-ear aid.

HEARING AID COMPONENTS

All hearing aids, regardless of type, utilize at least 4 major electrical components: microphone, amplifier, receiver, and power supply. Many hearing aids also include a number of other optional auxiliary circuits which increase the fitting flexibility and range of applications. Some of the optional auxiliary circuits utilize continuously variable, screwdriver-adjustable potentiometers for the audiologist and some of the optional circuits can be controlled by the patient. Examples of some of the auxiliary circuits include: (1) frequency response control (high frequency range and/or low frequency range); (2) maximum power output control; (3) compression control (input and/or output, etc.; (4) gain control; (5) telecoil; (6) directional versus omnidirectional microphone switch; (7) direct audio input connector/jack; and, (8) switching to select microphone input only, telecoil input only, or simultaneous microphone and telecoil input.

Microphones

The usual input to a hearing aid is through the microphone. Several types of microphones have been used with hearing aids across the years, including crystal, magnetic, ceramic, and electret. Crystal and ceramic microphones are relatively high-impedance microphones and were utilized most successfully with high-impedance vacuum tube amplifiers. The ceramic microphone was used for a period of time with solid-state amplifiers, but an impedance-matching circuit was necessary to match the high impedance of the microphone to the low impedance of the amplifier. Magnetic and electret microphones are low-impedance microphones and are used most successfully with the low-impedance, solid-state amplifier circuitry presently in use. Use of the electret microphone seems to be almost universal in hearing aid design in recent years. In comparison to other microphones available, the electret microphone has a smoother and broader frequency response, lower susceptibility to mechanical vibration and mechanical feedback, better sensitivity, and lower internal noise. Electret microphones are supplied to manufacturers in a number of different frequency responses and frequency ranges.

Electret microphones can be supplied in either the directional or omindirectional varieties. Directional microphones used in hearing aids are most efficient in picking up sound originating from in front and to the side of the hearing aid user and are designed to de-emphasize sound originating from behind the user. Many adult users prefer the directional microphone, particularly in noisy environments. Use of a hearing aid with a directional microphone for a school-age child must be given careful consideration. If it is important that the child be able to hear from all directions in the classroom, use of a directional microphone is probably contraindicated. If the unique arrangement of the classroom and the teaching style of the instructor are, however, such that it is usually significantly more important for the child to hear from the front than from behind, then a directional microphone should probably be considered and used on a trial basis.

Amplifiers

Amplifier circuit design seems to be in a continual state of flux with new innovations, refinements, and improvements appearing on a regular basis. Hearing aid amplifiers have all been solid state for several years. The particular technique utilized in the manufacture of present-day solid-state integrated circuit amplifiers has evolved into a highly reliable process which has enabled significant miniaturization of the amplifier block of hearing aids. The miniaturization of the amplifier has resulted in the availability of more room inside the hearing aid chassis for the addition of other controls, circuits, and options. Current amplifier design utilizes integrated circuitry with some "outboarding" to other circuits for accomplishment of specific functions.

All current hearing aid amplifiers are analog devices and operate using continuously variable amplification parameters. Manufacturers and developmental laboratories are currently in the process of designing digital hearing aids and appear to be on the threshold of introducing these devices to the market (Nunley, Staab, Steadman; Wechsler, & Spencer, 1983; Schneuwly, 1985). Digital signal processing in the prototype instrument described by Audiotone is accomplished by means of a central processing unit (CPU) which manipulates digitized data to obtain a result dictated by a software program. The introduction and ongoing development of digital hearing aid amplifiers will likely lead to a whole new concept of hearing aid design. One of the primary applications of the digital hearing aid seems to reside in its potential to effectively separate the signal from the noise, and the introduction of digital hearing aids is anxiously awaited by many educational audiologists who have struggled to deal with the effects of noise in classrooms for many years.

Hearing Aid Controls

Volume Control. Several circuit components have been designed to interact with the amplifier in controlling the hearing aid amplification characteristics. These include the volume control and the audiologist-adjustable gain, frequency response, output, and compression controls. The volume control wheel on a hearing aid simply controls the amount of gain provided by the hearing aid and is adjusted by the user to provide comfortable amplification. Care needs to be exercised in making sure that the hearing aid has sufficient gain without being turned fully on. Many hearing aids generate significant harmonic distortion when the volume control is turned to or near the "full on" position (Lotterman & Kasten, 1967). The volume control "taper" of hearing aids also needs to be checked in order that the user and/or the audiologist understand the operating characteristics of the volume control wheel. Although volume control wheel function has been improved in recent years, many volume control wheels on hearing aids are not linear. That is, a major portion of the increase in gain will be achieved by turning the volume control wheel only a portion of the total range, with very little change in gain occurring when the volume control is rotated in the upper part of the range. An idealized volume control taper function is shown in Part A of Figure 5-2 and a nonlinear volume control taper function is shown in Part B of Figure 5-2.

Gain Potentiometer. Auxiliary screwdriver-adjustable gain controls are also available on some post-auricle instruments. The audiologist-adjustable gain control is used to vary the limits of the patient-adjustable volume control wheel so that the volume control adjustments made by the user are in a maximally comfortable intensity range.

Frequency Response Potentiometer. Until recently, frequency response control of a hearing aid has, in essence, been accomplished by low-tone suppression. A "high-frequency emphasis" frequency response in a hearing aid is essentially accomplished by reducing the gain in the low frequencies, as shown in Part A of Figure 5-3, and not by actually increasing the gain in the high frequencies. The frequency response control is essentially a screwdriver-adjustable, high pass filter network which interacts with the amplifier in differentially controlling the difficulty of flow of electrical energy across frequency. Some recent post-auricle hearing aids also have a second frequency response control to reduce the amplification in the higher frequencies as shown in Part B of Figure 5-3. The frequency response control

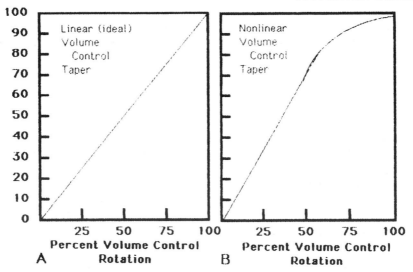

Fig. 5-2. Hearing aid volume control taper: (A) linear volume control taper, and (B) nonlinear volume control taper.

which reduces amplification in the higher frequencies can be very helpful in reducing acoustic feedback, but amplification often cannot be removed in the higher frequencies without materially altering speech discrimination or clarity of reception.

Maximum Power Output Potentiometer. The "maximum power output" control is a screwdriver-adjustable potentiometer used to limit the output of the hearing aid to a level below the uncomfortable listening level of the user. Many hearing aids have a control which varies gain and output together in an interactive way. Other hearing aids have independent gain and maximum power output controls.

Automatic Volume and Compression Controls. Many hearing aids also utilize some type of automatic volume control (AVC) or compression. While there are technical and design differences between automatic volume control and various compression systems, these terms are sometimes used interchangeably. These devices operate so that, as the output from (or input to) the hearing aid increases progressively, the amount of gain decreases progressively. In this way the user is protected from sound which approaches the uncomfortable listening level. Currently, there are several types of compressors available with varying claims made by those who advocate their use. There seem to be little objective data at the moment concerning which type of compression works best with different types and etiologies of hearing loss. It is generally agreed, however, that persons who have unusual difficulty

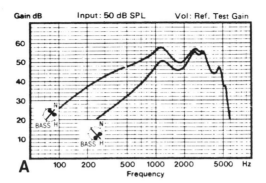

High Cut Control

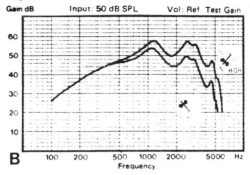

Fig. 5-3. Examples of effects of bass cut and high cut response potentiometers on hearing aid frequency response: (A) high frequency emphasis control, and (B) low frequency emphasis control.

tolerating loud sound (recruitment) should be fitted with a hearing aid incorporating an automatic volume control or compression circuit.

Receivers. All air-conduction hearing aids terminate the output in a hearing aid receiver or miniature speaker. The receiver functions to transduce the electrical signal received from the amplifier circuit back into an acoustical signal for delivery to the ear canal. The receiver is probably the weak link in hearing aids today. Current hearing aid receivers are "magnetic" and leave a little to be desired in terms of frequency response range and smoothness, sensitivity, and internal noise. Efforts are being made to develop a hearing aid receiver that will match the advantages of the electret microphone. Nevertheless, the magnetic receivers in current use are quite efficient when compensations are made in the circuitry which precedes them to account for their problems.

An alternate receiver in the form of a bone vibrator is available for use in special circumstances. Hearing aids designed to be terminated in bone-conduction vibrators are quite uncommon at present, but have definite applications. Basically, use of a bone-conduction hearing aid is indicated in cases where use of an air-conduction hearing aid is not possible or where use of an earmold is contraindicated. Examples of such cases include patients with congenital atresia or aplasia, patients with chronic and unresolved otitis media with discharge, and patients with allergic reaction to all the various chemicals used in the fabrication of earmolds. Bone-conduction vibrators are not as efficient as air-conduction receivers in delivering high-frequency energy to the cochlea, and bone-conduction receivers require considerably more power than do air-conduction receivers for equivalent auditory stimulation. Presumably for purposes of obtaining sufficient power to drive the bone-conduction vibrator, most bone-conduction hearing aids are of the body type. One advantage of a bone vibrator is that both cochleae are stimulated by a single vibrator. Only one microphone/amplifier/receiver system is used, however, in bone-conduction hearing aids and the stimulation of both cochleae from one bone vibrator cannot be considered as true binaural hearing, since subtle differences in phase, intensity, and spectral characteristics to the 2 ears are missing.

Optional Inputs.   During recent years, the flexibility of hearing aids has increased relative to the inputs they will accept. Current hearing aids will accept input from the hearing aid microphone, from the hearing aid induction (telephone) coil, from direct wire input from some external device such as a tape recorder or television, or from some combination of simultaneous inputs. The usual input from the built-in microphone of the hearing aid is sometimes referred to as the environmental microphone since it serves to pick up sound impinging on the microphone diaphragm originating from any source in the environment.

Many hearing aids can be switched from the microphone position to a telecoil position. The telecoil of a hearing aid is simply a magnetic induction coil which operates on the prinicple of transformer action. When the hearing aid is switched to the telecoil position, it will pick up only a fluctuating magnetic field generated by a device such as the telephone receiver held close to the ear. The telecoil of the hearing aid may also be used to pick up the magnetic field generated by the induction neck loop of an FM auditory training system as discussed in Chapter 7.

Several hearing aid models have been designed so that the microphone of the hearing aid can be used simultaneously with the induction coil. These hearing aids thus have a 3-position switch which allows the user to select the microphone (M), the telecoil (T), or both the microphone and telecoil (MT) positions. In the combined position, students can hear the primary speaker (teacher) through the FM system, but can also hear themselves and others through the environmental microphone. In addition to the M/T/MT selection possibilities, many hearing aids have a direct wire input jack. The direct wire input allows the user to plug the line output or auxiliary output of an external audio device such as a tape recorder or television set, or the direct wire output from an FM auditory trainer receiver, directly into the hearing aid, thus by-passing the distortion resulting from intermediate stages of transduction and also avoiding the reception of background noise originating in the environment. These input options allow students in the classroom to listen under many conditions at greatly improved speech-to-noise ratios and also to reduce the acoustic blurring resulting from adverse reverberation time common to many classrooms.

Power Supply. Every hearing aid must contain some kind of a power supply to provide the energy utilized in amplifying sound. Hearing aids worn on the person usually utilize a battery or cell. ("Cell" is the correct term. Use of the term "battery" is, however, more common and the 2 terms will be used interchangeably here.) Hearing aid batteries are provided in several common sizes and are made with several different chemicals. The 2 cells most commonly used in ear-level hearing aids at present are mercury or air-zinc. The cell used with most body hearing aids is the usual alkaline flashlight battery in the "AA" size. These cells provide a nominal voltage of approximately 1.35 volts. The mercury and air-zinc cells have a reasonably flat voltage decay curve and essentially allow the hearing aids in which they are used to operate in a consistent manner during the entire life of the battery. The zinc-air cells typically provide a battery life which is approximately twice that provided by mercury cells of the same size. The cost of a package of 6 mercury cells is usually reasonably equivalent to the cost of a package of 3 zinc-air cells. The cost for each hour of use is therefore approximately the same for the 2 types of batteries. The advantage of the zinc-air cells lies in the fact that they do not need to be changed as often as do the mercury cells.

Other available batteries include the silver-oxide cell and the nickel-cadmium cell. Silver-oxide cells are usually interchangeable with the same size mercury or zinc-air cells but provide slightly greater voltage and approximately 3 dB more gain in many hearing aids. Silver-oxide cells are currently considerably more expensive than either the mercury or zinc-air cells and do not provide battery life longer than that of the mercury cells. Nickel-cadmium cells are designed to be rechargeable and, while they have been intermittently available for several years, they have not come into common use. A new cell is currently under development; this battery uses lithium as its primary chemical. Lithium cells will have a nominal voltage of approximately 3 volts (twice the voltage of current hearing aid batteries), but commercially available hearing aids have not yet been designed which will utilize the higher voltage of the lithium cell. Lithium is a very lightweight material and the cells will have a shelf life of 5–10 years; longer than any other battery currently available.

Hearing aid batteries come in several sizes, including 675 (mercury or zinc-air), 76 (silver-oxide), 13 (mercury or zinc-air), 41 (mercury or zinc-air), and 312 (mercury or zinc-air). The majority of post-auricle hearing aids utilize the 675, although several models utilize the 41 cell. The majority of in-the-ear aids utilize the 13 size and the recently introduced in-the-canal hearing aids utilize the 312 cell. The vast majority of hearing aids utilize either the 675 or the 13 cell and these cells are available virtually all over the world. Some care needs to be exercised in making certain that batteries are purchased from suppliers who turn over their battery inventory often enough so that batteries are fresh. A battery tester can be a very helpful and inexpensive device to monitor battery voltage as part of an on-going program to assure optimum and consistent use of amplification in the school. Present hearing aids will not function when the battery voltage drops below approximately 0.9 volts.

Children sometimes experience difficulty in predicting when a hearing aid battery will be expended and, consequently, often find themselves with a dead battery and no replacement. For this reason, it is suggested that an extra battery or two be kept for each hearing-impaired child in each environment where the child spends appreciable time

Earmolds

With the exception of hearing aids utilizing a bone vibrator and certain tube-fitted hearing aids, all hearing aids must be coupled or fitted to the ear by means of some kind of earmold. Most earmolds are custom fabricated from an impression of the user's ear. The earmold serves several functions or purposes. First, the earmold is often used to effect some degree of occlusion or seal between the external auditory meatus and the outside air; the degree of occlusion depends to a major extent on the degree of hearing loss. The earmold essentially prevents amplified sound delivered to the external auditory meatus by the hearing aid from leaking or escaping to the outside air and re-entering the hearing aid microphone. When such a situation develops, the hearing aid will often whistle or squeal, a phenomenon referred to as "acoustic feedback". Acoustic feedback can usually be eliminated by changing the design or shape of the earmold and increasing the degree of occlusion, as discussed by Castleton (1983).

A second function of the earmold is to effect a comfortable and secure fit of the hearing aid to the ear. Individual ears are quite different and unique in size and shape and there is no such thing as a universal earmold. In order to assure comfort of the fit, earmolds are usually fabricated in special laboratories from individual impressions obtained by the audiologist.

A third function of an earmold is to modify the operating characteristics of the hearing aid. The frequency response of a hearing aid can be modified by changing such parameters as venting (low frequencies) and use of filters (mid frequencies), and by changing diameter, length, and shape of the tubing and sound bore (high frequencies). As shown by Killion (1981, 1982), the characteristics of a hearing aid can often be altered in very predictable ways by changing earmold parameters.

Considerable effort has been expended in recent years to develop earmold configurations to accomplish specific acoustic functions. Killion has developed several "tuned" earmolds to emphasize or de-emphasize the gain of the hearing aid in specific frequency regions. In addition, such innovations as the Libby horn (Libby, 1980, 1981, 1982; Libby, Johnson, & Longwell, 1981; Mueller, Schwartz, & Surr, 1981; Bornstein & Randolph, 1983), a series of Janssen molds (Janssen, 1984), and molds with continuous flow adaptation (Westone, 1984) have been introduced. Earmolds are supplied in a number of different configurations or styles from very small for people with slight and mild loss to quite large and bulky for people with severe hearing loss. A basic relationship exists between degree of hearing loss and the required bulk and occlusion of the earmold. Essentially, people with severe hearing loss require the most bulky and occluding earmolds to prevent acoustic leakage and the resulting feedback.

Any earmold style can be supplied with many different compounds. The most common compounds utilized in the fabrication of earmolds for hearing aids are lucite, various compositions of polyvinyl chloride (PVC), silicone, and polyethylene. Lucite is a hard, clear plastic and is the least expensive of the earmold materials. Lucite tends to generate an allergic reaction in some individuals and cannot be used by them. Futhermore, the hard lucite molds can result in a bruised or lacerated ear if the ear is bumped while the earmold is being worn, and such bumps are not uncommon in active children. The various compositions of PVC are relatively softer and more flexible than are the lucite molds and, for this reason, are safer for active children. PVC earmolds are relatively less likely to result in an allergic response than are lucite earmolds. The material least likely to result in an allergic response from the user is silicone. Silicone earmolds are relatively more expensive than other earmolds and are highly flexible, almost to the point of being difficult to insert. Silicone earmolds are very nonporous, so that it is difficult to glue a new tube into a silicone earmold. Tubes in silicone earmolds must be friction fitted or fitted with special cement and tubing. Polyethylene earmolds are also very hypoallergenic. These earmolds are usually white in color and are quite hard.

Earmolds are coupled to post-auricle and eyeglasses hearing aids by means of flexible tubing. The tubing is supplied in a number of different thicknesses and internal diameters as indicated by Blue (1979) in Table 5-1. The standard tubing is a "number 13," with an internal diameter of 0.076 inches. Earmold tubing tends to discolor, harden, and break over a period ranging from several months to 2 years. The tubing must be replaced when this occurs, and it is helpful for the educational audiologist to maintain a supply of replacement tubing and the various and sundry tools and cements needed to change earmold tubing when required.

Table 5-1.
Hearing aid tubing thicknesses

	Diameter in Inches	
Tubing Number and Size	internal diameter	outer diameter
9 standard	0.118	0.158
12 standard	0.085	0.125
13 standard	0.076	0.116
13 medium	0.076	0.122
13 thick	0.076	0.130
14 standard	0.066	0.116
15 standard	0.059	0.116
16 standard	0.053	0.116
16 thin	0.053	0.085

From Blue VJ. NAEL—An important part of the team. *Hearing Instruments,* 1979, *30*(12), 16. With permission.

HEARING AID CANDIDACY CONSIDERATIONS

Several factors must be taken into consideration in the process of deciding whether or not a particular student is a candidate for hearing aid amplification. The obvious factors relate to degree or magnitude of hearing loss and to the audiometric configuration. Less obvious factors, which are nevertheless important, include academic progress and achievement, social development, and speech and language development. It is the authors' collective opinion that serious consideration should be given to the child's potential in these areas and not simply to whether or not the student is performing at grade level expectations. If a child has a hearing loss and is not performing according to judged potential as determined by objective academic and psychological measures, hearing aid use should be considered.

Magnitude of Hearing Loss

The usual guidelines for determining candidacy based on magnitude of hearing loss for adults is usually something like; (1) 0–30 dB HL, usually no need for amplification; (2) 30–40 dB HL, borderline hearing aid candidate; (3) 40–55 dB HL, good benefit from hearing aid use; (4) 55–85 dB HL, greatest profit from hearing aid use; (5) 85–100 dB HL, hearing aid will probably provide some benefit; and, (6) 100+ dB HL, hearing aid use is seldom satisfactory (Berger & Millin, 1978).

While the above general guidelines are perhaps helpful in determining hearing aid candidacy, other factors such as demands on hearing and dependence on audition must be considered. A significant portion of the academic material presented in the classroom is presented orally and much of the learning which occurs in the schools takes place through audition. By and large, schoolchildren have extremely heavy demands placed on audition because of the nature of the classical instructional method used in most classrooms. Adventitiously hearing-impaired adults are often able to rely on past speech and language learning, acquired vocabulary, and auditory experience to the extent that they can "get by" in spite of some hearing loss. School-age children, on the other hand, are in the process of acquiring speech and language skills, acquiring vocabulary, and gaining auditory experience and learning. For these reasons, it seems that the intensity criteria utilized in determining hearing aid candidacy must be revised in the direction of fitting children with milder hearing loss than is the case with adults. It has been shown that many children with a hearing loss of 10–20 dB experience cummulative academic deficit, even when the hearing loss is intermittent, as is the case in children with recurrent episodes of otitis media. (See Chapter 4).

Audiometric Configuration

The audiometric configuration must also be considered in determining hearing aid candidacy. Generally speaking, it has been considered that flatter audiometric configurations are easier to fit than are sloping ones. The tendency seems to have been to not fit persons with mild high-frequency hearing loss when hearing through 1000 or 1500 Hz is well within normal limits. Speech science data from many sources indicates, however, that a major portion of information present in the spectrum of speech lies in the higher frequencies above 1000 Hz. It seems critical to provide children with mild high-frequency hearing loss with this high-frequency information by means of hearing aid amplification. Provision of amplification in the higher frequencies for these children seems particularly important when it is recognized that most ambient noise present in the environment is characterized by intensity in the lower frequency range and that the intensity of ambient noise in many classrooms is definitely sufficient to impair communicative efficiency. In classrooms where there is ambient noise, children with high-frequency hearing loss thus cannot rely consistently on the good hearing they have in the lower frequencies, due to masking from the low-frequency ambient noise. They cannot, futhermore, rely on hearing in the higher frequencies due to high-frequency hearing loss. Use of hearing aids to amplify in the higher frequencies may be of significant benefit to these children.

Binaural Amplification

In spite of the fact that there are several theoretical and practical factors to recommend use of binaural amplification, many audiologists still seem to be hesitant to recommend binaural amplification. After several years of experience fitting hearing aids on preschool and school-age children through many parent-infant programs in the nation (Clark & Watkins, 1985), it is abundantly apparent in a subjective way to all involved that most children with 2 aidable ears perform much better auditorally, academically, and socially with binaural than with monaural amplification. Callihan (1971), Ramaiya (1971), and Ross (1977) also provide data supporting the use of binaural amplification in children.

One probable advantage of binaural listening relates to localization of sound in 3-dimensional space. Localization skills are based on central nervous system comparisons of intensity, phase, and spectral differences received from the 2 ears. When only one hearing aid is used, the 2 ears are no longer reasonably well matched. Only when an aid is worn in each ear, so that hearing in the 2 ears is similar, is it reasonable to expect the brain to be able to utilize the small and subtle differences from the 2 ears in localizing sound. Strictly speaking, it is not necessary to be able to localize the source of sound in order to understand what is being said. On the other hand, localization skills add a dimension to audition which most listeners appreciate. There are, of course, reasons related to personal safety which suggest that attention should be given to optimizing localization skills in hearing-impaired listeners. Many hearing-impaired listeners rely at least to some extent on speechreading skills to supplement cues obtained from audition. Ability to localize the source of sound in 3-dimensional space helps to quickly find the speaker so that speechreading cues can be obtained.

A second possible advantage of binaural over monaural amplification relates to the ability of the auditory system to separate foreground from background and to hear against a background of noise (Carhart, 1965). In research and special auditory test applications, this phenomenon is referred to as the "masking level difference" and when the term is used in describing everyday listening situations, it is referred to as the "background squelch effect". It seems that when the signals arriving at the central auditory nervous system from the 2 ears are slightly different, the efficiency of the auditory system in separating two or more sound sources and identifying them as separate entities is improved. The signal-to-noise ratio seems to be improved internally through dichotic listening and the masking level difference can make a significant difference to speech discrimination in noisy listening conditions. Again, it is important to realize that the ambient noise levels in most typical classrooms leave a great deal to be desired.

A third and practical advantage of binaural amplification simply relates to the notion that, regardless of the source of the sound, one ear or the other (or both) is advantageously positioned so that the listener need not be continuously on guard to make sure the source of sound originates from the side on which the hearing aid is worn. Maintaining 2 hearing aids continuously in optimum working order is something of a major chore with some children. One possible advantage to fitting these children with 2 hearing aids is that, although both aids may not be working optimally on a continual basis, one aid or the other is likely to be operating appropriately so that the child has consistent amplification from at least one if not both ears.

There are, of course, isolated instances where use of binaural amplification is not practical or desirable. Hearing aids should not be fitted in ears with active middle ear disease with discharge, for obvious reasons. Binaural hearing aid use should be questioned when unaided audiometric data from the 2 ears are grossly discrepant. For example, fitting both ears of a person with excellent speech discriminatory capacity in one ear and very poor speech discriminatory capacity in the other ear can result in aided binaural hearing which is poorer than is aided monaural hearing when the hearing aid is in the ear with the better speech discrimination score. It is the authors' feeling, however, that, in all cases where both ears of a schoolchild are aidable, binaural amplification should be used until it is proven than monaural hearing aid use is more efficient.

Choice of Aided Ear in Monaural Fitting

In cases where it is determined that only one ear is to be fitted, the audiologist may use a series of untested axioms in making a decision as to which ear to fit. These axioms were presented by Watson and Tolan in 1949 and by Berger, Hagberg, and Rane in 1977. These axioms include: (1) Fit the ear with the best speech discrimination score; (2) Fit the ear with the greatest conductive component; (3) Fit the ear with the best tolerance for loud sound or the ear with the least recruitment; (4) If the better ear has a loss less than 55–60 dB HL (ANSI, 1969), in the speech frequencies, fit the poorer ear; (5) If the poorer ear has a loss greater than 70–80 dB HL (ANSI, 1969), fit the better ear; (6) Fit a healthy rather than an infected and draining ear; (7) If audiological findings are symmetrical, fit the ear which is not used with the telephone if the patient does not experience difficulty hearing on the telephone; (8) If audiological findings are symmetrical, fit the ear used with the telephone if the patient needs a telecoil for effective telephone communications; and (9) Fit the ear with the flattest audiometric configuration.

HEARING AID SELECTION/EVALUATION PRINCIPLES

After it has been determined that a child is, in fact, a candidate for a hearing aid system, decisions must necessarily be made concerning the most desirable set of electroacoustic parameters, input options, and earmold type. In many cases, the school-age child may not be able to provide reliable data from which valid decisions can be made. Maintaining interest and alertness during an entire hearing aid evaluation can be difficult when working with an adult and can be next to impossible when working with a child. It may be necessary to conduct the hearing aid evaluation/selection over several sessions rather than in one lengthy session in order to obtain appropriate co-operation from the child.

There are, of course, several different hearing aid evaluation philosophies which might be used in selecting a hearing aid for a school-age child. The goal of the present chapter is not to argue the relative merits of the various techniques. In fact, several of the techniques seem to have highly useful elements and there are circumstances where each can be advantageously used. Regardless of the method used in selecting a hearing aid for a hearing-impaired child, 2 principles must be kept in mind. First, it is somewhat unrealistic to expect aided thresholds of a hearing impaired client to be at "zero" dB HL at the conclusion of the fitting. Clients most often report that sound is uncomfortably loud when the gain of a hearing aid is turned up to provide "normal" aided thresholds. Several reports (Brooks, 1973; McCandless & Miller, 1972; Millin, 1965) indicate that aided thresholds which are approximately half to three-fifths the value of the hearing loss represent a more realistic goal. Libby (1985) noted that clients with mild to moderately severe sensori-neural hearing loss prefer a listening level close to one-third the value of the hearing loss. Second, care must be exercised in fitting children with severe and profound hearing loss with high-gain/power hearing aids. For these children, "more" is not necessarily "better". Hood and Poole (1966) indicated that: (1) The loudness discomfort level for both normal listeners and people with sensori-neural hearing loss is between 95 and 110 dB in 9 of 10 cases regardless of the magnitude of hearing loss; (2) Cochlear overload or degradation appears at about 100 dB SPL; (3) Significant temporary threshold shift (TTS) occurs when signal intensity exceeds approximately 100 dB SPL; and, (4) Care needs to be exercised to avoid risking additional permanent threshold shift (PTS) from signals that exceed these levels. Furthermore, studies dealing with electrophysiological auditory nerve potentials (Montandon, 1975) on both normal listeners and subjects with sensori-neural hearing loss evidence degradation of electrophysiological response at signal input levels above 115 dB SPL. Several reports (Bellefleuer & VanDyke, 1968; Derbyshire, 1977; Itakura, 1978; Jerger & Thelin, 1968; Macrae, 1968; Macrae & Farrant, 1965; Markides, 1976; Roberts, 1970; Ross & Lerman, 1967; Titche, 1977) indicate that hearing aids with high gain and output may result in additional hearing loss resulting from exposure to high-intensity sound.

Carhart/Northwestern Hearing Aid Evaluation Method

If the child is alert, has an appropriate attention span, and has reasonable linguistic competence, the traditional Carhart hearing aid evaluation process can be used (Carhart, 1946; Carhart 1950). Among other considerations, this method involves measurement of the aided speech reception threshold (SRT), aided speech discrimination in quiet, and aided discomfort level using several possible hearing aid systems or electroacoustic specification sets. The hearing aid is selected which provides the best overall aided performance when all measurements are considered together. The Carhart method utilizes widely available spondee and monosyllabic word list materials, the use of which may be questioned for younger children. Newer monosyllabic word lists such as the WIPI and NU-CHIPS (see Chapter 4) have been developed for use in measuring speech discrimination in children, however, and can be used as the stimulus materials in using the Carhart hearing aid evaluation method.

Synthetic Sentence Hearing Aid Evaluation Method

A second method which requires responses to speech material from the patient is espoused by Jerger and Hayes (1976). The Jerger method involves simultaneous presentation of a primary message consisting of 10 synthetic sentences and a competing message consisting of continuous discourse. The primary message (synthetic sentences) is presented repeatedly at 40 dB HL while the intensity of the competing message (continuous discourse) is varied to provide message-to-competition ratios (MCRs) between -20dB and +20dB. An articulation function is developed for each of several potentially useable hearing aids by plotting pecentage correct against the MCR. The hearing aid is chosen which provides the best MCR performance as indicated by the articulation function curve.

Computational Methods

In cases where it is difficult to obtain valid verbal responses from children, the audiologist may wish to use one of the computational hearing aid selection procedures, at least as a starting point. While several computational methods have been presented, the method which is probably most widely used is the Berger method (Berger, Hagberg, & Rane, 1977). Some computational hearing aid evaluation methods utilize a computer in accomplishing the necessary calculations (Mason & Popelka, 1982; Skinner, Pascoe, Miller, & Popelka, 1982; Starkey, 1984) and others utilize a computer and probe microphone assembly for accomplishing real ear measurements (Libby, 1985; Nielsen & Rasmussen, 1984).

Berger Computational Method

The computations required in the method described by Berger, Hagberg, and Rane (1977) can be accomplished quickly without the aid of computational equipment, although a hand-held calculator is helpful. The Berger method assumes a standard set of conditions and does not take into account the unique dimensional character of the specific client's external ear or the unique characteristics of the earmold to be used. The Berger method is essentially based on the observation that most hearing aid users set the volume control of their hearing aid(s) so that aided pure-tone thresholds are approximately half to three-fifths the value of the hearing loss as indicated by the pure-tone threshold measured under earphones (Brooks, 1973; Mc-Candless & Miller, 1972; Millin, 1965). The divisor utilized in the computation at each frequency is chosen so as to take into account: (1) the differences between standard HA-1/HA-2, 2cc coupler measurements and real ear measurements; and, (2) the shape of the long-time average speech spectrum. Attention is also given to limiting the maximum power output of the hearing aid(s) to a level below the uncomfortable listening level of the client and to limiting the output in the low frequencies so as to reduce the discomfort from amplified low-frequency noise (Griffing & Hinz, 1972; Kretchmer, 1974; McCandless & Miller, 1972) and to reduce decrease in speech intelligibility resulting from spread-of-masking (Egan & Hake, 1950; Harbert & Young, 1965; Jerger, Tillman, & Peterson, 1960; Rittmanic, 1962; Sweetow, 1977; Viehweg, 1968.

CID Computer-Assisted Method

The Central Institute for the Deaf (CID) computer-assisted hearing aid evaluation program, (Mason & Popelka, 1982; Popelka & Engebretson, 1983; Skinner, Pascoe, Miller & Popelka, 1982) takes into account the unique properties of the patient's external ear and the unique characteristics of the earmold to be used. Basically, the program involves computation of an articulation index (AI) value for the hearing aid system under consideration (French & Steinberg, 1947; Kryter, 1962; ANSI, 1969). The computations are rather involved and time-consuming if accomplished by hand. For this reason, a computer program has been written to: (1) accept the audiometric data obtained from the patient; (2) accept the electroacoustic data from the hearing aid under consideration; (3) make the necessary conversions and corrections from the different intensity references utilized in obtaining the data; and, (4) compute the AI value.

Computation of the AI yields a number relating to the proportion of the long-time average speech spectrum between 250 and 6000 Hz which is more intense than the pure-tone thresholds and less intense than the uncomfortable listening level. Classic speech science studies (Dunn & White, 1940) have shown that a 30-dB intensity range encompasses most of the intensity range between the minimum intensity of normal conversational speech and the maximum intensity of normal conversational speech in each of several frequency bands between 250 and 6000 Hz. If the speech minimums in each of the several frequency bands exceed the respective pure-tone thresholds, and if the speech maximums in each of the several frequency bands do not exceed the uncomfortable listening level for the respective frequency bands, then the contribution to intelligibility contributed by each band will be maximal and the AI value will be "unity" or 1.0.

The overall goal is to center the long-time average speech spectrum around the Most Comfortable Listening Level (MCL), at the same time making sure that the speech minimums exceed the pure-tone thresholds and that the speech maximums do not exceed the Uncomfortable Listening Levels (UCL). Ordinarily, the AI is expressed as a number between 0.0 and 1.0. For purposes of the CID hearing aid program, however, the AI value is multiplied by 100 in order to obtain the percentage of the speech spectrum falling in the dynamic intensity range between the pure-tone thresholds and the uncomfortable listening levels of the client. It is important to realize that the percentage score yielded by the program is an AI value and is not a predicted speech discrimination score. It is possible, however, using a nomogram presented in the 1962 Kryter article on the AI, to obtain the speech discrimination score that would be predicted for a normal listener using the same amplification system.

Use of the computer-assisted hearing aid evaluation program requires a standard audiometer with sound field speakers, an electroacoustic hearing aid test system, and a Hewlett-Packard Model 85, or Apple Model IIe computer. In order to utilize the program, certain minimal data must be entered into the computer. These data include pure-tone thresholds obtained under earphones; most comfortable listening levels for pure tones between 250 and 6000 Hz obtained under earphones; uncomfortable listening levels for pure tones between 250 and 6000 Hz obtained under earphones, pure-tone sound field tresholds (using either one third octave bands of noise or frequency-modulated pure tones) for frequencies between 250 and 6000 Hz obtained from a trial hearing aid; and gain and Maximum Power Output (MPO) of the trial hearing aid (ANSI, 1976) as used by the patient during the trial.

Once sound field pure-tone thresholds have been obtained using the trial aid coupled to the ear with an actual earmold, the audiologist can compute the AI and display the data graphically. The audiologist can then determine what changes need to be made in the electroacoustic parameters (gain and MPO) of the hearing aid in order to optimize the fitting by positioning the amplified speech spectrum between pure-tone tresholds and uncomfortable listening levels. The changes can be entered and the effects of the changes evaluated by re-computing the AI. The process of changing electroacoustic parameters of the hearing aid can be repeated until the audiologist is satisfied that an optimum fit has been achieved. The computer can then be asked to provide a listing of recommended 2cc coupler gain and MPO values with the hearing aid set to the comfort setting.

The computer-assisted program is based solidly on speech science data which have been in existence for decades. The direct application of these data to hearing aid selection is of sufficiently recent origin, however, that validating evidence of the method is still somewhat lacking. Although minor changes may need to be made in the ultimate hearing aid fitting, the com-puter-assisted hearing aid evaluation technique outlined by CID certainly represents a highly useful point of departure in selecting hearing aids for children.

VALIDATION OF APPROPRIATENESS OF HEARING AID FITTING

The best hearing aid in the world is the one that is worn. A hearing aid obviously will not provide listening assistance to a user if it is not worn. Several factors may be offered as explanations or excuses as to why hearing aids are sometimes not used consistently. Some of these may relate to social stigma and vanity. Before such factors are accepted as possible reasons for hearing aid rejection, however, the audiologist must rule out discomfort arising either from poorly fitting earmolds or from overamplification and must rule out inability to hear because of underamplification.

If social stigma or self-consciousness are problems in early stages of hearing aid use, support, reassurance, and gentle insistence must be provided by all educational personnel interacting with the hearing-impaired child. The educational audiologist must play a major role in helping the hearing-im-paired child accept and adjust to the hearing aid(s) when hearing aid use is indicated. It has been the authors' experience over several years that, with proper orientation and support, hearing-impaired children typically prefer to wear their hearing aids in the classroom rather than be without the enhanced listening ability the aids provide.

Benefit from hearing aid use must be demonstrated in one or more of several ways before the fitting can be considered successful. The educational audiologist must obtain unaided and aided audiometric data and must com-pare these results for children, their parents, and concerned educational personnel. Parents, teachers and other educational personnel, and significant others must report on observed changes in auditory and verbal behaviors. One of several tools which may be used to help these people to quantify their observations is the "Significant Other Assessment of Communication Scale" developed by Schow and Nerbonne (1982).

In addition to the above, pre-fitting and post-fitting growth rates can be obtained from objective measures of academic, social, and emotional skills. In short, everyone associated with the child must be convinced that amplifi-cation will be of benefit and, furthermore, must be committed to do whatever is necessary to make certain the hearing aids are worn. Downs (1967, 1971) has presented several very helpful suggestions for establishing hearing aid use in children. The suggestions are, for the most part, common-sense applications of behavior modification principles and will not be enumerated here.

HEARING AID MANAGEMENT

It is one thing to select and fit an optimal hearing aid system and to establish appropriate habits and patterns of use. It is quite another thing to assure that the hearing aid(s) function according to factory specifications continuously over months and years of vigorous use. Incriminating data have been presented in several reports over many years concerning the appalling number of hearing aids, worn by children in various educational settings, which do not work appropriately (Bess, 1977; Coleman, 1972; Gaeth & Lounsbury, 1966; Porter, 1973; Schell, 1976; Zink, 1972). These studies have involved several geographical locations and several educational/clinical settings, and have encompassed many years. They constitute an indictment against all those involved in managing the hearing aids of hearing impaired children. Educational audiologists, audiologists, teachers, and parents must all accept responsibility. Hearing-impaired students who are old enough to be responsible for their own welfare must also accept partial responsibility for wearing "dead" hearing aids and hearing aids with dead batteries. The situation is particularly discouraging when one considers the wealth of information available concerning the management and maintenance of hearing aids (Bill Wilkerson Hearing and Speech Center, 1974; Clark & Watkins, 1985; Craig, Sins, & Rossi, 1976a, 1976b; Design Media, 1980; Downs, 1967; Downs, 1971; Gauger, 1978; Hanners & Sitton, 1974; Kweskin, Bartlett, Kalbfeisch & Stone, 1981; Mynders, 1979; Ross & Giolas, 1978; Rubin, 1975). The above references contain excellent information concerning hearing aid use and care. While it is not the goal of the present chapter to outline the details of hearing aid care and troubleshooting, several general principles must be seriously considered with regard to achieving optimal and consistent amplification.

Training the User and the User's Parents/Guardians

The authors have found that, with proper encouragement and training, older schoolchildren will report sudden changes in hearing aid amplification. The subtle deterioration in acoustic performance which occurs over time is, however, more difficult for hearing-impaired children to identify than is a sudden change. In cases where children cannot be depended upon to report changes in the quality of sound received through the hearing aid, some other person must accept responsibility for checking the hearing aid on a daily basis. Daily listening checks are strongly recommended, since judgments relative to possible malfunction of the hearing aid(s) are made on the basis of comparisons with an internal reference obtained from listening to the hearing aid(s) on previous occasions. Ideally, the parent or guardian will receive training from the educational audiologist and will accept the responsibility for performing a listening check of the hearing aid on a daily basis.

Training Educational Personnel

Unfortunately, not all parents or guardians will accept the responsibility for performing the daily listening check and, in these cases, someone in the schools such as a teacher or an aid must be trained by the educational audiologist to accomplish the task. Ideally, the educational audiologist would perform the listening checks. Many educational audiologists, however, do not see each hearing-impaired child at school on a daily basis and, in fact, many schools do not have the services of an educational audiologist. In these cases, the school speech and hearing clinician must assume the functions of an educational audiologist in assuring that daily listening checks are performed and that the hearing aid(s) function appropriately over time.

Electroacoustic Evaluation

In addition to the daily listening checks, each hearing aid should be given a complete electroacoustic evaluation on a periodic basis. It is recognized that most school districts do not have an electroacoustic hearing aid analysis system. A great many clinical audiologists involved in the dispensing of hearing aids, however, have electroacoustic analysis systems and are willing to aid the educational audiologist in analyzing the hearing aids of schoolchildren on a periodic basis. Most university audiology training programs also have the necessary instrumentation. The electroacoustic evaluation should include measurement of gain, MPO, frequency response, harmonic distortion, telecoil sensitivity, internal circuit noise, volume control taper, compressor function, and battery current drain. It is suggested that these measurements be obtained using the ANSI-1969 protocol and also that they be obtained at the "use" setting.

At a minimum, the electroacoustic evaluation should be conducted prior to the beginning of each school year and again midway through the year. Any hearing aid reported by a hearing-impaired child or by a responsible adult to have changed in amplification characteristics or to be obviously malfunctioning should immediately be evaluated electroacoustically and sent for repair if found to perform unsatisfactorily. Ideally, a loaner hearing aid should be fitted to the hearing-impaired child while the hearing aid is being repaired and some effort should be made to obtain a supply of loaner hearing aids. Various service organizations have been known to donate or contribute to the cost of obtaining loaner instruments for use by schoolchildren while their hearing aids are being repaired.

Common Problems and Troubleshooting

Earmold Blockage. Many of the hearing aid problems which develop with ongoing hearing aid use are preventable or solveable without sending the hearing aid to the manufacturer for repair. Before a hearing aid is sent to the manufacturer for repair, several common trouble spots should be checked. It is not uncommon for hearing aid earmolds to become clogged with cerumen, foreign materials, or condensed droplets of water. In these cases, the hearing aid will sound dead because sound cannot penetrate the blockage. If the hearing aid is found to function when the earmold tubing and/or earhook are removed, the audiologist can be assured that a blockage exists in the tubing or the earmold and steps should be taken to remove the blockage using a fine probe and either air or water pressure. In some cases, it may be necessary to extract and replace the tubing in order to remove the blockage.

Changing Earmold Tubing and Earhooks. Earmold tubing tends to discolor, lose flexibility, shrink, and eventually crack with age. When it hardens to the point that the fit is uncomfortable, when it comes loose from the earmold, or when it cracks or breaks, the earmold tubing must be replaced. The educational audiologist should maintiain a supply of common sizes of tubing (sizes 12–16) and the cement necessary to replace the tubing in earmolds. The replacement process is greatly simplified if the tubing is ordered "pre-bent" and "quilled" from the earmold lab.

Earhooks of behind-the-ear hearing aids occasionally become stripped and/or loose where they screw/attach to the receiver nozzle. Screw-on earhooks are inexpensive and can be replaced simply by removing the old earhook and screwing on a new one. Screw-on earhooks can be obtained from any one of several firms which supply hearing aid parts and accessories (Hal-Hen, for example). Other hearing aid models use friction-fitted earhooks which are pressed on or snapped into place. These are usually available from the respective hearing aid manufacturer.

Problems With Moisture. Excessive moisture from perspiration and/or high humidity can result in hearing aid malfunction or intermittency. A dessicant pack of silica gel may be placed, together with the hearing aid, in a sealed plastic container to keep the aid free of moisture or to dry it once it has been dampened. Silica gel dessicant packs have been developed specifically for this purpose and are available from hearing aid parts and accessories supply houses such as Hal-Hen in New York. The dessicant packs can be used over and over and can then be recycled by heating in the oven at 350°F for a few hours.

Battery Contacts and Battery Freshness. Battery freshness and function seem to raise continual problems unless the user has access to a hearing aid battery tester. A hearing aid will not function with less than approximately 0.9 volts and a battery tester is very helpful in assessing whether or not the battery is functionally dead. A hearing aid obviously will not function with a dead battery and the solution to the problem should be equally obvious. A hearing aid battery testing device is a must for anyone who deals with assessing hearing aid function on a regular basis. Proper attention must be paid to observing proper battery polarity. A remarkable number of hearing aid users come in for help when the only problem is that the battery is in upside-down. On occasion, the battery compartment and the battery leads can become corroded and coated to the point that a poor electrical connection is achieved between the battery and the battery contacts. The battery contacts can be cleaned with a pencil eraser.

Acoustic Feedback. Acoustic feedback can also present problems for the hearing aid user and other people in the immediate environment. The first step in correcting a problem relating to feedback is to assess the source of the acoustic leak. The acoustic leak may occur between the earmold and the ear canal from a poorly fitting earmold. The acoustic leak may also result from a vent which is too large, from a loose connection between an external receiver and an earmold, from loose or broken earmold tubing, from a loose or broken earhook, or from loose or disconnected tubing between an internal receiver and the nozzle. The audiologist must simply work from the earmold backward, closing off the earmold, tubing, and earhook, until the feedback is eliminated. For example, if the feedback is eliminated when the audiologist closes off the sound bore and vent of the earmold, the feedback can be assumed to be the result of a poorly fitting earmold or a vent which is too large. If the feedback is still present when the sound bore and vent are occluded, then the source of the feedback must necessarily be between the earmold and the hearing aid. The next step is to remove the tubing from the earhook, occlude the end of the earhook, and again check for feedback. If feedback is not present with the earhook occluded, the source of the feedback is the tubing. If the feedback is still present, the source of the feedback is between the earhook and the hearing aid. The next step is to remove the earhook and occlude the receiver nozzle. If the feedback is thereby eliminated, the source of the feedback is the earhook. If the feedback is not eliminated, the source of feedback is internal and the hearing aid should be sent to the manufacturer for repair. Once the source of the feedback is determined, the audiologist can take steps to correct the problem. It may be necessary to occlude the earmold vent, build up the earmold, or obtain a new and tighter-fitting one. It may also be necessary to replace the tubing and/or the earhook if these are the source of the problem.

Hearing Aid Repair

On occasion, it will be necessary to return a hearing aid to the manufacturer or other facility to be cleaned, repaired, reconditioned, and returned to original manufacturer specifications. The usual turnaround time required for hearing aid repair and reconditioning is between 1 and 2 weeks. Most dispensing audiologists and other dispensers will supply the user with a loaner aid while the hearing aid is away for repair. The cost of repair of an instrument is relatively constant from manufacturer to manufacturer and the aids are returned with at least a 6 month warranty. The manufacturers usually repair the obvious problems, recondition the hearing aid(s), and accomplish preventative maintenance while the hearing aids are in the laboratory.

Hearing Aid Insurance

A final comment should be made regarding hearing aid insurance. School-age children are prone to be very hard on hearing aids due to their high activity level and lack of maturity. It is not unusual for school-age children to lose hearing aids or to damage them severely in any of a number of ways. For this reason, parents and/or guardians should seriously consider obtaining hearing aid insurance, particularly during the first year of use. Insurance for a hearing aid is between 15 and 25 dollars a year, depending on the manufacturer or insurance company. If the family decides to purchase insurance, it is usually necessary to do so within 10 days of the date of the hearing aid fitting.

REFERENCES

American National Standards Institute. American National Standard methods for the calculation of the articulation index. American National Standards Institute, New York: ANSF 1969.

American National Standards Institute. Specification of hearing aid characteristics, American Standard S3.22-1976. New York: ANSI, 1976.

Bellefleuer P A & VanDyke R C. The effect of high gain amplification on children in a residential school for the deaf. *Journal of Speech and Hearing Research.* 1968, *11,* 343–347.

Berger K W, Hagberg E N, & Rane R N. *Prescription of hearing aids: Rationale, procedures and results.* Kent, Ohio: Herald Publishing House, 1977.

Berger K W & Millin J P. Hearing aids. In D Rose (Ed.). *Audiological assessment* (ed. 2). Englewood Cliffs, N.J.: Prentice-Hall, 1978.

Bess F H. Condition of hearing aids worn by children in a public school setting. In F B Withrow (Ed.), *The condition of hearing aids worn by children in a public school program.* (Report No. (OE) 77-05002, Grant No. OEG-4-71-0060). Washington, D.C.: U.S. Department of Health, Education, and Welfare, Office of Education, 1977.

Bill Wilkerson Hearing and Speech Center. *Changing sounds* (Slide-tape program). Nashville, Tenn., 1974.

Blue V J. NAEL—An important part of the team. *Hearing Instruments,* 1979, *30,* 16.

Bornstein S P & Randolph K J. Research on smooth, wideband frequency responses: Current status and unresolved issues. *Hearing Instruments,* 1983, *34,* 12–16.

Brooks D. Gain requirements of hearing aid users. *Scandinavian Audiology,* 1973, *2,* 199–205.

Callihan V A. A comparison of binaural and monaural hearing aid performance of preschool children. Unpublished master's thesis, Vanderbilt University, 1971.

Carhart R. Tests for selection of hearing aids. *Laryngoscope,* 1946, *56,* 680–694.

Carhart R. Hearing aid selection by university clinics. *Journal of Speech and Hearing Disorders,* 1950, *15,* 106–113.

Carhart R. The background squelch effect: A phenomenon of binaural listening. Paper presented at the American Speech and Hearing Association, Chicago, November, 1965.

Castleton L. NAEL; Fitting facts, Part IV, Feedback—not the problem, the solution. *Hearing Instruments,* 1983, *34,* 24–26.

Clark T C & Watkins S. *The Ski*Hi model, programming for hearing impaired infants through home intervention, home visit curriculum.* (ed. 4). Logan, Utah: Ski*Hi Institute, 1985.

Coleman R F. *Stability of children's hearing aids in an acoustic preschool* (Final Report, Project No. 522466, Grant No. OEG 4-71-0060). Washington, D.C.: U.S. Department of Health, Education, and Welfare, Office of Education, 1972.

Craig H, Sins V, & Rossi S. *Hearing aids and you.* Beaverton, Ore.: Dormac, Inc., 1976a.

Craig H, Sins V, & Rossi S. *Your child's hearing aid.* Beaverton, Ore.: Dormac, Inc., 1976b.

Cranmer K S. Hearing Aid Dispensing-1984, *Hearing Instruments,* V. 35, No. 5, May 1984, 9–15.

Derbyshire J O. A study of the use of high power hearing aids by children with marked degrees of deafness and the possibility of deterioration in auditory acuity. *DSH Abstracts,* 1977, *17,* 1 (For *British Journal of Audiology:* 1976, *10*(3), 74–78.)

Design Media. *Hearing aids: A daily check* (filmstrip or sound/slide program). Oakland, Calif.: Design Media, 1980.

Downs M P. The establishment of hearing aid use: A program for parents. *Maico Audiological Library Series,* 1967, 4 (report 5).

Downs M P. Maintaining children's hearing aids: The role of the parents *Maico Audiological Library Series,* 1971, 10 (report 1).

Dunn H K & White S D. Statistical measurements on conversational speech. *Journal of the Acoustical Society of America,* 1940, *11,* 278–288.

Egan J P & Hake H W. On the masking pattern of a simple auditory stimulus. *Journal of the Acoustical Society of America,* 1950, *22,* 622–630.

French N R & Steinberg J C. Factors governing the intellibility of speech sounds. *Journal of the Acoustical Society of America.* 1947, *19*(1), 90–119.

Gaeth J H & Lounsbury E. Hearing aids and children in elementary schools. *Journal of Speech and Hearing Disorders,* 1966., *31,* 283–289.

Gauger J S. *Orientation to hearing aids.* Washington, D.C.: The Alexander Graham Bell Association, 1978.

Griffing T S & Hinz. Beware the pain threshold! *National Hearing Aid Journal* 1972, *25,* 7, 28, 32.

Hanners B A & Sitton A B. Ears to hear: A daily hearing aid monitor program. *The Volta Review,* 1974, *76,* 530–536.

Harbert F & Young I M. Spread of masking in ears showing abnormal adaptation and conductive deafness. *Acta Otolaryngology,* 1965, *60,* 49–58.

Hood J & Poole J. Tolerable limit of loudness: Its clinical and physiological significance. *Journal of the Acoustical Society of America,* 1966, *40*(1) 47–53.

Itakura S. Changes of hearing thresholds in children wearing hearing aids. *DSH Abstracts,* 1979, *19,* 3. (for *Audiology Japan:* 1978, *21*(3), 143–149).

Janssen G V. *Cookbook of tube fitting for hearing aids.* 830 N.W. 10th Street, Oklahoma City, Oklahoma, 73106, 1984.

Jerger J & Hayes D. Hearing aid evaluation: Clinical experience with a new philosophy. *Archives of Otolaryngology.* 1976, *102*, 214–225.

Jerger J & Thelin J. Effects of electroacoustic characteristics of hearing aids on speech understanding. *Bulletin of Prosthetics Research,* Fall, 1968, pp. 159–197.

Jerger J F, Tillman T W, & Peterson J L. Masking by octave bands of noise in normal and impaired ears *Journal of the Acoustical Society of America,* 1960. *32*, 385–390.

Killion M C. Earmold options for wideband hearing aids. *Journal of Speech and Hearing Disorders,* 1981, *46*(1) 10–21.

Killion M C. Transducers, earmolds, and sound quality consideration. In G A Studebaker & F H Bess (Eds.) *The Vanderbilt hearing aid report.* Upper Darby, Penn.: Monographs in Contemporary Audiology, 1982.

Kretchner L. Evaluation procedures for adults. In Donnelly K (Ed.) *Interpreting Hearing Aid Technologies.* Springfield: Charles C. Thomas, 1974.

Kryter K D. Methods for the calculation and use of the articulation index. *Journal of the Acoustical Society of America,* 1962, *34*(11), 1689–1697.

Kweskin S, Bartlett P C, Kalbfleisch K E, & Stone R I. *Hearing aids, a guide to their wear and care.* Daly City, Calif.: PAS Publishing, 1981.

Libby E R & Smooth. Wideband hearing aid responses—The new frontier. *Hearing Instruments,* 1980, *10*, 12–18.

Libby E R. Achieving a transparent, smooth, wideband hearing aid response. *Hearing Instruments,* 1981, *32*, 9–12.

Libby E R. In Search of Transparent Insertion Gain Hearing Aid Responses, in Studebaker G A & Bess F H. *The Vanderbilt Hearing Aid Report,* Monographs in Contemporary Audiology, 1982, 112–123.

Libby E R. State of the art of hearing aid selection procedures. *Hearing Instruments,* 1985, *36*(1) 30–38; 62.

Libby E R, Johnson J H, & Longwell T F. Innovative earmold coupling systems. Chicago, Ill.: Zenetron, 1981.

Lotterman S H & Kasten R N. The influence of gain control rotation on nonlinear distortion in hearing aids. *Journal of Speech and Hearing Research,* 1967, *10*, 593–599.

Macrae J H. TTS and recovery from TTS after use of powerful hearing aids. *Journal of the Acoustical Society of America,* 1968, *43*(6) 1445–1446.

Macrae J H & Farrant R H. The effect of hearing aid use on the residual hearing of children with sensori-neural deafness. *Annals of Otolaryngology, Rhinology, and Laryngology,* 1965, *74* 409–419.

Mahon W J. The Year of the ITE: 1984 U.S. Hearing Aid Sales, *The Hearing Journal,* 1984, *37*(12) 7–11.

Markides A. The effect of hearing aid use on the user's residual hearing. *DSH Abstracts,* 1977, 17, 3. (For *Scandinavian Audiology:* 1976, *5*(4) 205–210.)

Mason D & Popelka G R. *Program for hearing aid selection and evaluation: User's guide for Phase IV.* St. Louis, Mo.: Central Institute for the Deaf, 1982.

McCandless G A & Miller D L. Loudness discomfort and hearing aids. *Natural Hearing Aid Journal,* 1972, *25*, 7; 28; 32.

Millin J P. Speech discrimination as a function of hearing aid gain: Implications in hearing-aid evaluation. Unpublished Master's Thesis, Western Reserve University, 1965.

Montandon P B. Auditory nerve potentials from ear canals of patients with otologic problems. *Annals of Otolaryngology, Rhinology and Laryngology,* 1975, *184*(1), 165–168.

Mueller H G, Schwartz D M, & Surr. R K. The use of the exponential horn in an open mold configuration, *Hearing Instruments,* 1981, *10*, 16–18.

Myndes J M. A beginning hearing aid maintenance program. *Hearing Aid Journal,* 1979, *32*(7), 9–41.

Nielsen H B, & Rasmussen S B. New aspects in hearing aid fittings. *Hearing Instruments*, 1984, *35*(1) 18–20; 48.

Nunley J, Stabb W, Steadman J, Wechsler P, & Spencer B. A wearable digital hearing aid. *The Hearing Journal*, 1983, *36*, 29–34.

Popelka G R, & Engebretson A M. A computer-based system for hearing aid assessment. *Hearing Instruments*, 1983, *34*(7), 103–105.

Porter T A. Hearing aids in a residential school. *American Annals of the Deaf*, 1973, *118*, 31–33.

Ramaiya J J. A study of binaural hearing aid performance. Unpublished master's thesis, Vanderbilt University, 1971.

Rittmanic P A. Pure tone masking by narrow-noise bands in normal and impaired ears. *Journal of Auditory Research*, 1962, *2* 287–304.

Roberts C. Can hearing aids damage hearing? *Acta Otolaryngologica*, 1970, *69*, 123–125.

Ross M. Binaural versus monaural amplification for hearing impaired individuals. In F H Bess (Ed.), *Childhood deafness: Causation, assessment and management*. New York: Grune & Stratton, 1977.

Ross M & Giolas T G. Issues and exposition. In M Ross & T G Giolas (Eds.), *Auditory management of hearing-impaired children*. Baltimore: University Park Press, 1978.

Ross M & Lerman J. Hearing aid usage and its effect upon residual hearing. *Archives of Otolaryngology*, 1967, *86*, 639–644.

Rubin M. *All about hearing aids*. Washington, D.C.: The Alexander Graham Bell Association, 1975.

Schell Y S. Electro-acoustic evaluation of hearing of hearing aids by public school children. *Audiology and Hearing Education*, 1976, *2*, 7; 9; 12; 15.

Schneuwly D. Digital technology, the hearing aid and computer fittings. *Hearing Instruments*, 1985, *36*, 16–17; 62.

Schow R L & Nerbonne M A. Communication screening profile: Use with elderly clients, *Ear and Hearing*, 1982 *3*, 135–147.

Skafte M. Hearing Health Care Market Potential of the 80's, Part 1: Hearing Aid Market Analysis. *Hearing Instruments*, 1984, *35*, (5), 16–20.

Skinner M W, Pascoe D P, Miller J D, Popelka G R. Measuresments to determine the optimal placement of speech energy within the listener's auditory area: A basis for selecting amplification characteristics. In G A Studebaker & F H Bess (Eds.), *The Vanderbilt Hearing Aid Report*. Monographs in Contemporary Audiology, 1982, 161–169.

Starkey Laboratories. Model CA1, Computerized fitting analyzer, description/specification sheet. Minneapolis: Starkey Laboratories, 1984 (advertising brochure).

Sweetow R W. Temporal and spread of masking effects from extended low frequency amplification. Journal of Audiological Research, *1977* 17, 318–321.

Titche L L, Windrem E O, & Starmer W T. Hearing aids and hearing deterioration. *Annals of Otolaryngology, Rhinology and Laryngology, 1977, 86*(3) 357–361.

Viehweg S H. Differential effects of signal and noise filtering on speech intelligibility in sensorineural hypacusis. Unpublished doctoral dissertation, Northwestern University, 1968.

Watson L & Tolan T. *Hearing tests and hearing instruments*. Baltimore: Williams and Wilkins, 1949.

Westone Laboratories. Product manual/descriptive literature, for earmold supplies/tools and earmold impression materials, 1984.

Zink G D. Hearing aids children wear: A longitudinal study of Performance. *The Volta Review*, 1972 *74*, 41–51.

Frederick S. Berg

6
Listening and Speech Skills

This chapter describes a basis for and specific programs for assisting most hard-of-hearing students and many near-deaf students to develop listening and speech skills. Such skills are highly useful for both interpersonal communication and development of reading and writing skills. Lundsteen, who has been a leader within the National Council of Teachers of English, points out that a listening curriculum should be integrated early within the total language arts curriculum. The same could be said about a speech curriculum.

> Why put listening first in the language arts? For one reason, listening is the first language skill to appear. Chronologically children listen before they speak, speak before they read, and read before they write . . .Reading may depend so completely upon listening as to appear to be a special extension of listening. What child does not read a selection better after hearing and talking about it?. . . .Writing in turn, is both directly and indirectly dependent upon listening because of its relation to speaking on one hand and to reading on the other. (Lundsteen, 1971, p. 3).

In this chapter, emphasis will be given initially to basic information about listening and speaking and then to specific programs and procedures. There will be descriptions of sound and hearing, learning and perception, current communicative methodologies for the hearing impaired, and many popular or promising listening and speech programs. Both developmental and refinement programs will be covered. The role of self instruction and training sources for teachers and parents will also be discussed.

BASIC LISTENING AND SPEECH CONSIDERATIONS

Unfortunately, listening and speech training for the hearing impaired is neglected in both the regular schools and in special schools for the hearing impaired. In regular schools, few special direct services of any kind are available for the hearing impaired. In the great majority of special schools, signs are used, and neither listening nor speech is given the emphasis needed.

A systematic listening and speech program requires both tests and tasks. The baseline performance of the child should be assessed so that training can be intelligently planned. Infant and preschool programs and school programs are needed to close listening and speech gaps as much as possible. Speech training particularly requires a long-term sustained effort, especially for children with severe and profound hearing loss. Listening and speech training are appropriately provided in tandem, giving emphasis to speech perception and then to speech production.

Visual listening or speechreading (lipreading) training is often needed in addition to auditory training. A listening test, therefore, should assess both visual and auditory speech perception in addition to auditory-visual speech perception. The assessment should encompass samples of speech stimuli within a child's language repertoire. A listening test should provide options for measuring word perception, sentence perception, and message perception. The subtests administered may vary from one hearing-impaired child to another, and from one age to another age with the same child.

A speech test is also given if the hearing-impaired child has a speech problem in addition to an auditory or visual listening problem. The purpose of a speech test is to identify and assess each vocal, prosodic, and articulatory speech target in error. The young child, particularly the youngster with a severe or even greater hearing loss, will need longitudinal speech assessment. Initially, just the most basic speech targets need to be assessed and later more and more complex speech targets may be assessed.

It is not known to what extent auditory or auditory-visual stimulation should be used in listening training. Unisensory auditory stimulation has been recommended to ensure that the hearing-impaired child develop a predominately auditory orientation rather than a reliance on lipreading or sign communication (Erber 1982; Pollack 1985; Wedenberg 1954). Bisensory stimulation is recommended because of the combined roles of audition and vision for linguistic and cognitive development. Sanders (1982 pp. 374–379), believes that training should proceed from highly redundant to less redundant conditions by systematically reducing auditory and visual clues in various life situations. However, Ling (1976) states:

In order to develop ability to perceive many of the acoustic cues that are required for adequate auditory-visual speech reception, prior and parallel training in speech reception through audition alone should be provided (p.51).

Minimum criteria for effective spoken communication may be described. The hearing-impaired child should be able to say familiar words or sentences so that the clinician can understand 90 percent of them. This child should also be able to recognize 90 percent of these same speech stimuli under the audiovisual (AV) condition when spoken by the clinician. The room should be a quiet and nonreverberant space. The child and clinician should be 3–5 feet from each other, facing each other. The child should also be able to communicate with the clinician as effectively at a distance of 12–15 feet in a noisy or reverberant room when personal FM equipment is used. The alternative to effective listening and speech skills for the hard of hearing or near-deaf child may be the use of signs for communication, a less functional option in general society (Ross, 1982).

SOUND AND HEARING

Sound and hearing are fundamental to listening and learning to speak. Sound is defined as vibrations or propagated vibrational energy which can be heard. Sound has intensity, duration, and frequency dimensions.

Intensity of sound can vary over a range of 10 billion watts—from .00000000000000001 watts for each square centimeter (0 dB) to .0000001 watts for each square centimeter (100 dB). No wonder hearing level or hearing loss is not figured on a percentage basis! Intensity is, instead, expressed in decibels (dBs) based on powers of 10, on a logarithmic rather than a linear scale. The child's detection level is defined by an intensity level where that child is just aware of the presence of a sound that, to the child, is very soft. Normally this is 0 dB.

Frequency of sound varies from 16 cycles each second (Hertz—Hz) to many thousands of Hertz. A pure tone has a single frequency or vibrational rate. A speech sound is complex in that it has a great many simultaneously occurring frequencies. Each vowel and consonant has a unique pattern of frequencies and intensities. The pitch of a voice is determined by the lowest frequency component. A characteristic pitch or fundamental frequency for a child is 260 Hz, compared with 230 Hz for an adult female and 130 Hz for an adult male. Vowels generally contain more low-frequency components than do consonants. The three vowels /oo/, /ah/, and /ee/ and the two consonants /sh/ and /s/ vary in overall frequency pattern from low to high and are representative of the 40 vowels and consonants of speech. They comprise Ling's (1981) Five Sound Test.

Duration of sound refers to the time in milliseconds required to produce a vowel or consonant or parts of speech sounds. The sounds of speech vary in duration as well as in intensity and frequency pattern. They also vary in durational characteristics according to where they occur in words and sentences. Duration provides valuable cues for perception of speech prosody as well as speech articulation.

The hearing losses of many children must be extreme before sounds that are detected cannot be discriminated or recognized following training. The intensity, frequency, and duration phenomena provide perceptible cues for many children with even 100-dB hearing loss. In contrast, there are chil-

Table 6-1.
Sample utterances made by Sven at 6-month intervals from
12–36 months

Month	Sample Utterance
12	Mama, bowwow
18	uppa go
24	I want more.
30	Let Sven go down and iron.
36	When Louis is big like me, I'll be bigger.

From Berg F. Language development. In F Berg & S Fletcher (Eds.), *The hard of hearing child.* New York: Grune & Stratton, 1970, 11–124.

dren with only moderate hearing loss who have difficulty discriminating speech, particularly in the presence of noise. Each child's hearing capabilities, including detection and discrimination capacities, need to be assessed sufficiently to determine the potential of the auditory sense for learning communication skills. Diagnostic listening training is essential!

LEARNING AND PERCEPTION

The greater the hearing loss, ordinarily the longer a child requires to learn to listen and speak. For example, a child with a moderate loss may learn twice as fast as a child with a severe loss and eight times as fast as a child with a profound loss (Prescott & Turz, 1975). This assumes that these 3 hypothetical children wear appropriate hearing aids.

Listening, language, and speech training should begin as soon as possible in the life of a hearing-impaired child. One reason for beginning early is to prevent the possible imperfect development or deterioration of the hearing sensory mechanism due to lack of early stimulation. A second reason involves taking advantage of the early years of life in which language develops very rapidly. A third reason for beginning early is the desire not to disturb the synchrony of perceptual and motor development, which proceeds on schedule despite missing sensory information. Hearing-impaired children often become used to a world without hearing and must be retrained to reorganize their developing world models of perceptions and conceptions (Boothroyd, 1982, Ross, 1982).

Audition is critically important for language and conceptual development as well as for listening and speech development. Table 6-1 illustrates one normal hearing child's unusually rapid development of language and concepts, from use of single words at 12 months to employment of complex sentences at 36 months (Berg, 1970).

A case study of the perceptual learning of auditory, visual (speechreading), and electrovisual speech cues by a college student with over a 100-dB hearing loss demonstrates the importance of early auditory training. This student had previously attended an elementary public school program for the hearing impaired and a regular secondary school. He had been given special training in speech and language through a visual-oral approach and had a high motivation to speak and to improve his speech. Given auditory training at age 22, he quickly showed he could recognize the vowels and consonants of speech, particularly with visual or electrovisual support. He could repeat isolated phonemes as well as words, although he had much more difficulty recognizing sentences, a difficulty at least partially attributable to his limited syntactical competence. Also, the auditory training did not change his voice quality, which was harsh. It may be hypothesized that had an auditory-oral approach had been an integral part of this student's education from the preschool years onward, he might have attained voice, speech, and language skills that approached normality.

The advantage of starting early with listening training is exemplified in the story of Staffan Wedenberg, who had an audiogram similar to that of the case just described. (Wedenberg & Wedenberg, 1970). Staffan's detection threshold was 75 dB at 500 Hz, 95 dB at 1000 Hz, and "no response" at 2000 dB and above. His father, Erik, who pioneered auditory training in Sweden, correlated spectrographic and audiometric information to predict the consonants, vowels, and diphthongs Staffan might identify auditorily if sound were appropriately intense and if sufficient training were given. Erik initiated auditory training immediately after confirmation of hearing loss or at age 2½ years. A chronology of events and programming derived from a case history of Staffan Wedenberg is presented in Table 6-2.

Watkins (1984) recently compared hearing-impaired children who had received home intervention, including listening training, before they were 30 months of age to a similar group which had received it after 30 months of age and to another group which had not received any training. Language, academic achievement, psycho-social functioning, and parent attitude measures were obtained when these children were 6–13 years of age. Analyses of covariance, multiple comparison procedures, and effect size analysis were used to determine group differences. Analyses revealed that home-intervention children performed better than no-home-intervention children with respect to the majority of dependent variables. Slight favoring of early over late intervention and preschool over no preschool children was also apparent.

COMMUNICATION METHODOLOGIES

The majority of young hearing-impaired children in special schools and programs for the deaf throughout the United States can probably develop language and conceptual skills through a combination of auditory and visual

Table 6-2.
Age and Significant Events and Communicative Achievements
of Staffan Wedenberg

Age (years)	Significant Event or Achievement
2½	Parents recognize that Staffan is at least profoundly hearing impaired. They begin a unisensory auditory program of speech stimulation.
3⅔	Staffan now functions as a hard-of-hearing child. He has progressed through stages of sounds awareness, vowel perception, word perception, and sentence perception by use of audition only.
4	Staffan says his first sentence spontaneously, "Toto, utta, aj-aj." The sentence is elicited by a fear that his dog Tutta will be trampled by a horse.
4½	Staffan learns to read or to associate sounds and letters.
5	He achieves a spoken or expressive vocabulary of 400 words, forms many sentences, and begins to use verbs in the perfect and future tenses. He speaks spontaneously but defectively, uses no signs, and is uninhibited, finding friends among normal-hearing children his own age.
6½	His spoken vocabulary includes at least 600 words.
7	Staffan enters ordinary school and later transfers to a class for hard-of-hearing children. He also learns to read piano music. In addition, he requests that his name be changed to Douglas because he cannot hear Staffan well. He also begins wearing a series of innovative hearing aids and receives speech instruction.
14	His vocabulary approaches normal. He has received better than passing grades in most of his subjects taken in junior high and high school.
17	Staffan's vocabulary compares favorably with requirements for intelligent adults.
30	Having completed a degree in forestry some years earlier, he speaks fluent Swedish and English. On a trip to the United States, his speech is as intelligible as that of his father.

From Berg F. *Educational audiology: Hearing and speech management.* New York: Grune & Stratton, 1976, 98. With permission.

speech cues delivered through appropriate amplification and with the assistance of well-trained clinicians. This majority can detect sound up to 2000 Hz and should be taught to auditorially discriminate and recognize most of the English vowels and consonants. They should also be taught to perceive a significant percentage of words and sentences through vision or lipreading alone. The combination of auditory and visual cues provides sufficient sensory input to enable many children to use speech rather than signs in learning the English language. Schools or programs for the hearing impaired in the United States usually do not provide the hearing-impaired child with sufficient motivation to learn speech, with resultant detrimental consequences to listening and speech skills, and oral language development.

In a recent investigation, Geers, Moog, and Schick (1984) studied the acquisition of spoken and signed English by a sample of 327 children with profound hearing loss, from auditory oral (AO) and total communication (TC) programs across the country. Each child was tested on the Grammatical Analysis of Elicited Language—Simple Sentence Level (GAEL-S), which measures production of selected English language structures. Percentage correct scores for the oral productions of TC children were substantially below scores for their manual productions and below the oral scores of AO children on all grammatical categories sampled on the GAEL-S. The data indicate either that spoken English does not develop simultaneously with manually coded English or that efforts were not made in the TC sample above to ensure that signs were correlated with oral production.

The Cued Speech method is a third communicative option in the education of hearing-impaired children. In contrast with TC, this method inherently requires that the hands correlate with speech. It is only when the hand cue and lip position are correlated that a speech sound is recognized. With TC, the sign conveys meaning independent of speech that is being used. Nicholls and Ling (1982) describe Cued Speech in some detail.

In Cued Speech the consonants are cued by eight hand configurations and the vowels by four hand positions. Diphthongs are cued by gliding from the position of the initial to the final vowel nucleus. In running speech, the consonant-vowel hand cues are coarticulated, in a one-to-one relationship with the syllables of the language. A sender is able to transmit the cues in real-time synchronously with speech, thus conveying a visual analog of the syllabic-phonemic-rhythmic patterns of spoken language (p. 262)

In a study of the use of Cued Speech for the reception of spoken language, 18 children with hearing losses from 97 to 122 dB averaged 95 percent recognition of key words in sentences. They had been taught through the use of Cued Speech for at least 4 years. Nicholls and Ling (1982) concluded that Cued Speech: (1) is compatible with simultaneous auditory processing; and, (2) merits more widespread use as an oral option for those children who are deaf, near-deaf, or who do not progress adequately in more conventional oral programs.

Neither the TC nor Cued Speech (CS) methods may be needed by children who can perceive through a combination of auditory and speechreading cues at least 90 percent of the language they can express and comprehend. It is well worth the effort to provide auditory and visual (speechreading) training to all hearing-impaired children to determine whether they can achieve this criterion. Educational programming should be designed to provide an AO track for these functionally hard-of-hearing children in addition to the TC or CS option for functionally deaf children. From a long-range economic standpoint, it is going to be more cost-effective to provide at least AO and TC or CS options. From a social view, a child is going to benefit from listening and speech training, notwithstanding the communicative option being used in the home or school setting.

LISTENING AND SPEECH PROGRAMS

Parent/Infant Auditory Program

One of the most successful handicapped-education projects recently supported by the federal government has been Project SKI*HI Outreach, which assists in establishing home intervention programming for hearing-impaired infants and their families throughout the United States (Clark & Watkins, 1985). The demonstration base of the project is the state of Utah, where ongoing intervention is being conducted in more than 100 homes in both urban and rural localities under the name Parent Infant Program (PIP), administered by the Utah State School for the Deaf. Under PIP or SKI*HI Outreach, children with substantial hearing impairment are identified early in life, evaluated extensively, and their parents given psychological support and special training through weekly home visits until program goals are reached. Three home-visit programs are provided to parents and children in each home: (1) hearing aid: (2) auditory, and, (3) communication and language. Total Communication (TC) is also provided for children who do not evidence auditory language development solely through audition. Hearing aids are used with all children except the totally deaf. The home auditory program has recently been revised to incorporate early speech activities along with the auditory training activities it had emphasized previously.

The revised SKI*HI home auditory program includes 4 developmental phases and 11 skills. (The age of the child upon entry into the program and the amount of hearing loss are among factors that determine the actual time spent in each phase.) The 11 listening and speech skills to be developed are: (1) attending; (2) early vocalizing; (3) recognizing; (4) locating; (5) vocalizing with inflection; (6) hearing at distances and levels; (7) producing vowels and consonants; (8) environmental discrimination and comprehension; (9) vocal discrimination and comprehension; (10) speech sound discrimination and comprehension; and, (11) speech use.

These 11 skills are not necessarily all developed in sequence or developed at all. For example, discriminating and comprehending environmental sounds is not an essential prerequisite to discriminating and comprehending speech sounds. And, too, certain children with hearing loss may not acquire locating skill or true directional hearing.

Parent and child goals are set up for each listening and speech skill. Strategies for reaching them are also included. Parents are taught to train their children and to check progress in reaching these skills.

For a young hearing-impaired child to discriminate, comprehend, imitate, and meaningfully use speech ordinarily requires a year or more of full-time hearing aid use and auditory-oral stimulation. Once the child can listen in quiet, mild or strong distractions are introduced to prepare that child for more difficult listening situations. The program is flexible so that children of varying ages and hearing loss, upon entry, can be individually accommodated.

Pollack Mobilizing Residual Hearing

The auditory program of Project SKI*HI has been greatly influenced by the pioneering work of Erik Wedenberg (1954) and Doreen Pollack (1985). The progress of Staffan, Erik's son, has been described previously. Both Wedenberg and Pollack advocate and practice unisensory auditory approaches. Videotapes available from the Alexander Graham Bell Association for the Deaf show Pollack at work with parents and hearing-impaired children.

The Rules of Talking

A contemporary of Pollack, Kay Horton, describes the auditory language stimulation that accompanies specific methodology for the development of auditory skills. Horton (1973) stated that most young hearing-impaired children could learn aural and oral language through auditory stimulation, particularly when using binaural hearing aids. Twenty-seven suggestions, called "rules of talking", were classified under 5 headings and are specified below.

How to Get and Maintain the Child's Attention.
1.   Get down on the child's level, as close to his ears as possible.
2.   Let your face and your voice tell your child that what you are doing is interesting and fun.
3.   Let the child actively participate. Language is best learned while doing.
4.   Tune into the child. Talk about what interests him.

What to Talk About.
1.   Talk about the here and now.
2.   Talk about the obvious.
3.   At times, talk for the child.
4.   Put the child's feelings into words.

How to Talk to a Child Who Doesn't Yet Have Spoken Words.
1.   Everything has a name. Use the name.
2.   Use short, simple sentences.
3.   When you use single words, put them back into a sentence.

4. Use natural gestures when you talk.
5. Tell, then show the child what you are doing.
6. Use repetition. Say it again and again.
7. Give the child a chance to show that he understands.

How to Help a Child Use His Voice to Make Sounds.

1. Imitate the child's repeated movement and add voiced sounds to go along with the movement.
2. Vary the sounds you make to the child. Make it interesting for him to listen.
3. Give the child a chance to use his voice. Be a listener as well as a talker.
4. Imitate the sounds the child makes.
5. Reward the child when he uses his voice.

How to Talk when the Child Begins to Use Words.

1. Reward the child when he attempts to say a word.
2. Repeat the child's word and put it into a sentence.
3. When the child uses telegraphic speech, repeat his thought in a complete sentence.
4. Expand the child's vocabulary by adding new words.
5. When the child uses incorrect language or speech, repeat it correctly.
6. Let the child hear new sentence forms.
7. When the child expresses an idea, expand his thoughts by adding new information.

—Lillie, Head Teacher

Ling Developmental Speech Program

Observers note that the earliest vocalizations of a hearing-impaired infant are natural and accompanied by reflexive speech breathing patterns. Through early intervention, it is often possible to capitalize upon and reinforce these vocal and rhythmic skills (Boothroyd, 1982). With or without early intervention, a speech acquisition program for a severely or profoundly hearing-impaired child requires informed, systematic, and sustained effort over many years (Ling, 1976, p. 9). Speech, however, is an area in which many teachers of the hearing-impaired feel inadequate. In a popular book (1976) and in plan (1978a) and record (1978b) manuals, Dan Ling outlines the developmental stages and steps for teaching speech skills.

Ling also details spectrographic data for each of the consonants, vowels, and diphthongs as the basis for careful exploitation of residual hearing. While he emphasizes the importance of early intervention, he has trained even deaf adults to talk functionally.

Ling (1976) notes that speech must be developed at both imitative (phonetic) and spontaneous (phonologic) levels. He describes the levels and skills

Table 6-3.
Seven parallel phonetic and phonologic stages for speech
acquisition in hearing-impaired children.

Stage	Phonetic	Phonologic
I.	Vocalizes freely and on demand.	Uses vocalization as a means of communication.
II.	Bases of suprasegmental (duration, intensity, pitch) patterns.	Uses different voice patterns meaningfully.
III.	All diphthongs and vowels with voice control.	Uses different vowels to approximate words.
IV.	Consonants by manner with /i/, /u/, and /a/.	Some words said clearly and with good voice patterns.
V.	Consonants by manner and place.	More and more words said clearly and with good voice patterns.
VI.	Consonants by manner, place, and voicing.	Most words said clearly and with good voice patterns.
VII.	Initial and final blends.	All speech intelligible and voice patterns natural.

required: (1) producing orosensory-motor speech patterns; (2) auditorially differentiating one's own speech patterns; (3) listening to others' speech patterns and comparing them with one's own speech patterns; (4) comprehending the meaning of others' speech; and, (5) using one's own speech meaningfully. Ling (1976) notes that in order for speech to be functional, the child must speak reflexively so that complete attention can be given to what is being said. Phonetic drill is used to compensate for previously missed prelinguistic utterance practice, basic to normal spoken language acquisition. Phonologic activities are required to transfer imitative speech skills into meaningful utterances. Ling avocates using touch and vision or speechreading in addition to audition.

In the Ling program, the skills to be learned are sequenced within the 7 stage model of speech acquisition shown in Table 6-3. Vocal skills are initiated in the first stage, prosodic in the second, and the many articulatory skills in the third through seventh stages.

Ling (1976) has also developed a comprehensive speech evaluation for a hearing-impaired client. This evaluation includes (1) an oral peripheral examination of the structure and functioning of the speech organs; (2) a preliminary phonological evaluation of a 50-utterance tape sample; and, (3) a determination of whether many essential speech subskills are present in a client's phonetic repertoire. In the phonetic evaluation, a clinician indicates whether a series of target behaviors is produced consistently, inconsistently, or not at all. The phonetic evaluation encompasses vowels and dipthongs in isolation, simple consonants and word-initial blends in 3 syllables apiece, and word-final blends in syllables.

A unique SRAP marking system is also incorporated to varying extents in Ling's phonetic evaluation. The "S" means that a client can sustain a single syllable containing the target behavior at loud, quiet, and whispered levels. The "R" is marked when the syllable can be repeated at a rate of 3/second. "A" is checked when the same syllable can be alternated with any other syllable at the same rate. The "P" is checked when the client can vary pitch over 8 semitones while producing the syllable containing the target behavior. Ling emphasizes that the absence of one or more of these subskills interferes with the feed-forward demands inherent in fluent speech.

Each stage of the Ling program is divided into a specific number of speech targets. In turn, each speech target is subdivided into subskills. In Stage VI, for example, the fricatives /s/ and /z/ are differentially taught. Initially, these are taught in isolation. Then they are taught following vowels /u/, /a/, and /i/ in vowel consonant (VC)syllables. The client is then required to produce each of these syllables repeatedly. These fricatives are then held for at least 3 seconds in the same syllables. The /s/ and /z/ targets are then produced in the intervocalic position of contexts like /izi/ initially with each syllable equally stressed and thereafter with one vowel stressed and the other not. The /s/ and /z/ are then produced in the initial position of single syllables like /so/ and /zu/. Then /s/ and /z/ are taught in such syllables as /pasapasa/ and /wiziwizi/. Finally, these fricatives are produced in final, medial, or initial position of syllables using the 8-semitone pitch variation.

Speech Evaluation of the Deaf

In addition to the Ling evaluations, other tools are being used to evaluate the speech of hearing-impaired children. Two evaluative tools that have been used considerably with deaf children and young adults respectively are: (1) Magner (1972) speech intelligibility sentences developed at the Clarke School for the Deaf; and, (2) the Rainbow Passage used at the National Technical Institute for the Deaf (Subtelny, Orlando, & Whitehead, 1981).

The Magner test requires a child to orally read short sentences which are recorded and played back to auditors. Each syllable of each sentence in a set is scored for understandability. Scores are converted to percentages and plotted on a cumulative speech record kept on each child. The graphs are filed and periodically inspected for identification of problems and record of progress. The test is to be administered in October and April of each year. Two problems with the Magner test are its poor reliability and its being an oral reading test and therefore limited to use with older children.

The NTID test is a part of a Speech and Voice Characteristics of the Deaf Package. This package "has been developed to teach a diagnostic system for identifying and rating deviant speech and voice characteristics of the hearing impaired and to provide practice in using the speech and voice diagnostic system" (Subtelny, The Orlando, & Whitehead, 1981). The authors point out that this package is needed, since it is very difficult to accurately describe connected speech, a necessity for formulating an individualized education plan of speech training for any person with impaired hearing.

> The teachers, who assume specified responsibilities for training speech of the hearing impaired, must develop a high degree of auditory skills so they can analyze and describe the speech, voice and language problems presented. Such description is not a simple task, nor can requisite skill be achieved without experience, usually accumulated over many years (subtelny, Orlando, & Whitehead, 1981, p. 35).

Over 800 recorded samples from NTID students were analyzed to develop the training package, which is valid, reliable, and effective in training diagnostic skills. Ten speech and voice characteristics were identified: intelligibility, pitch register, pitch control, rate of syllable production, control of air expenditure, prosody, tense/harsh voice quality, breathy/weak voice quality, phyaryngeal resonance and nasal resonance distortion. A 5 point scale was developed to rate the deviation of each of the 6 speech characteristics and 4 voice qualities. Audio cassettes, answer keys, learner response sheets, and student performance record forms are included with explanatory material of the training package.

SPEECH REFINEMENT PROGRAM

The great majority of hearing-impaired children are hard of hearing rather than deaf. A hard-of-hearing child perceives speech more adequately than does a deaf child and consequently develops speech to a fuller extent with less special effort. Many hard-of-hearing children, however, still have speech deficits that need to be overcome through special training.

The Precision Speech Package of Berg and Child (in press) includes 133 vowel, diphthong, and consonant programs that can be used to refine the speech articulation of hard-of-hearing children and even older deaf youngsters who have developed prerequisite speech and voice skills. A test is administered to determine errors. Training may proceed from speech targets that are ordinarily developed earliest to those usually developed last. The Ling subskills for a target in error may be included or bypassed if the more basic vocal and prosodic targets are intact in a child's phonetic and phonologic systems.

Table 6-4 provides an index to the 133 articulation programs. The vowel

Table 6-4.

Index of 133 articulation targets included in the Berg
speech test and tasks

Program	Context	Program	Context	Program	Context	Program	Context
1	-i-	34	str-	67	-gz	100	bl-
2	-I-	35	spl-	68	-blz	101	br-
3	-e-	36	spr-	69	-ndz	102	-b
4	-ɛ-	37	-s	70	-pḷz	103	-bɚ
5	-æ-	38	-sṇ	71	-tṇz	104	-bḷ
6	-u-	39	-sp	72	-ʒ-,-ʒ	105	d-
7	-ʊ-	40	-sk	73	dʒ	106	dr-
8	-o-	41	-st	74	-dʒ	107	-d
9	-ɔ-	42	-ks	75	p-	108	-ld
10	-a-	43	-ts	76	pl-	109	-nd
11	-ʌ	44	-ps	77	pr-	110	-ṇd
12	-aɪ-	45	-stɚ	78	-p	111	-dɚ
13	-aʊ	46	-nts	79	-mp	112	-dḷ
14	-ɔl	47	-ʃ	80	-lp	113	-bd
15	-ɪu-	48	-ʃ	81	-pḷ	114	g-
16	f-	49	tʃ-	82	-mpḷ	115	gl-
17	fr-	50	-tʃ	83	t-	116	gr-
18	fl-	51	-ntʃ	84	tr-	117	-g
19	-f	52	h-	85	-t	118	-gd
20	-fs	53	v-	86	-nt	119	m-
21	-ft	54	-v	87	-tḷ	120	-m
22	-fts	55	-vz	88	-tṇ	121	n-
23	θ	56	-vd	89	-pt	122	-n
24	θr	57	ð-	90	-kt	123	-ŋ
25	-θ	58	-ð	91	k-	124	-ŋz
26	s-	59	z-	92	kl-	125	l-
27	sk-	60	-z	93	kr-	126	-l
28	sm-	61	-lz	94	kw-	127	r-
29	sn-	62	-mz	95	-k	128	-ɚ
30	sp-	63	-nz	96	-kɚ	129	-rn
31	st-	64	-zd	97	-kl	130	-rk
32	sl-	65	-bz	98	-ŋk	131	w-
33	sw-	66	-dz	99	b-	132	hw-
						133	j-

and diphthong targets are listed first and afterwards the consonant targets.
All targets listed have at least 4 referent words that can be pictured for training.
Some targets have as many as 12 such words.

During testing or training the accuracy of each articulation target is rated
by the clinician on a 4-point scale. A "1" is marked for a precise production,
a "2" for a light or mild distortion, a "3" for a moderate or severe distortion,
and a "4" for a profound distortion, a substitution, or an omission. A target

with a bull's-eye, an inner ring, and an outer ring may be used to portray judgment of accuracy of response. A "1" is placed in the bull's-eye, a "2" in the inner ring, a "3" in the outer ring (still on target), and a "4" off target. An on-target response is still recognized as being the target sound.

As the test is being administered, the clinician points to a picture of a word that includes the speech target and says the word so the client can hear and see it said. The client then repeats the word while the clinician listens and watches. The clinician then records a 1, 2, 3, or 4, and further information if desired. These numbers are recorded on a summary form that classifies the correct and error productions and provides an easy reference for making training recommendations.

During training with a target sound, the clinician gives instructions, records accuracy, and provides feedback on correctness of each response. The target sound is shaped in certain word stimuli of a particular program and tested for generalization in other word stimuli of the same program. Shaping is done initially under the echoic condition and then under picture, printed word, and printed sentence conditions. If following the McLean (1967) procedure, combined conditions are also included. Fading can also be employed, in which fewer and fewer preceding condition stimuli are paired with current condition stimuli as a target sound is mastered. Pass and fail criteria can also be arbitrarily set up to facilitate articulation mastery and transfer among stimuli. Once mastered in the articulation program, the corrected target response can be practiced in self-generated sentences using program words, and monitored in conversation (Bokelmann, 1973).

VOCAL SCOPE

Precise speech accuracy for a child who does not hear accurately may depend upon the addition of an electrovisual speech aid like the Vocal Scope shown in Figure 6-1. As the clinician speaks precisely and carefully into the microphone, the speech model is shown as a radial pattern. Each speech sound change has a unique radial pattern change that corresponds to the acoustic input. For a voiceless sound, the clinician can be the model for the client and both will produce the same radial pattern for a given speech target if both speak precisely. For a voiced sound, the same precision will produce different radial patterns if the clinician and client use different vocal pitch or quality or amount of nasality. In the latter instance, the client has to be his own model. When he produces a response that is desirable, the corresponding radial pattern becomes the model to duplicate.

Berg (1976) used radial patterns in addition to auditory, speechreading, and tactile speech cues to shape the articulation of a child with a profound hearing loss. After 10 training sessions, Berg judged that the child had im-

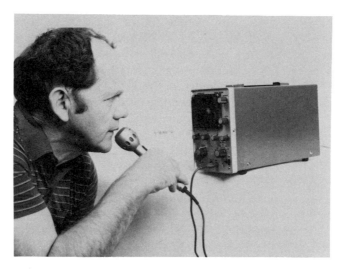

Fig. 6-1. Vocal Scope with radial pattern for /s/ sound. Compliments of Amera Incorporated, Logan, Utah.

proved accuracy of articulation of 36 vowel, diphthong, and consonant targets in error. Figure 6-2 shows baseline versus final measurements of accuracy of articulation for this child.

AUDITORY SKILLS PROGRAM

The listening and speech of hearing-impaired children will be enhanced if auditory skills are developed beyond those fundamentally developed during the early years of life. The Auditory Skills Instructional Planning System (ASIPS) of Los Angeles County Schools provides a curriculum specifically for hearing-impaired students from 4–12 years old with losses greater than 55 dB. Field studies indicate that the objectives and instructional activities may be applicable for older children as well. The philosophy behind this early school program is described below.

> Auditory training is a method for increasing the use of the auditory channel in concept development and language learning. Auditory experiences are constantly occurring: auditory training can make these experiences meaningful. New concepts may be enriched by focusing attention on the auditory experience as well as the other sensory experiences of seeing, touching, smelling, and tasting. Planned individual instruction and informal group instruction are needed to provide effective auditory training (ASIPS, p. 3.)

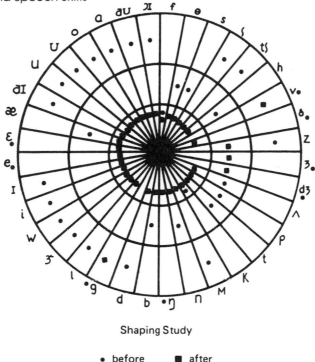

Shaping Study

• before   ■ after

Fig. 6-2. Shaping study. Baseline and final measure of accuracy in the articulation of 36 vowels, diphthongs, and consonants by a deaf child. • = before ■ = after.

The ASIPS curriculum provides training in: (1) detection of, attention to, and differentiation among messages; (2) recalling, in proper sequence, one or more messages; (3) using hearing to monitor one's own speech; and, (4) demonstrating any of the above skills under various listening conditions. The curricular goals are to assist the student to: (1) improve in comprehension of spoken language; and, (2) increase linguistic fluency and speech intelligibility.

The curricular materials of this program include the Test of Auditory Comprehension (TAC), the Auditory Skills Curriculum manual, the Audio Worksheets, Media for Auditory Training, and videocassette demonstrations. The TAC is standardized for children from 4 to 12 years old with moderate through profound hearing losses. It should be administered in a sound suite or quiet room under standardized procedures. Ten subtests are included, covering discrimination, memory-sequencing, and figure-ground (O dB signal-to-noise ratio) items in that order.

Normative data on TAC performance for students who have moderate, moderate-severe, severe, and profound hearing losses are included. Age of child is not a determining factor. Baseline and probe tests can be administered to an individual hearing-impaired student for comparison with one of these norms. Results of the TAC can be used to place the student in the auditory skills curriculum at an appropriate point.

The auditory skills curriculum provides terminal performance objectives and intermediate performance objectives (IPOs). A complete outline of the objectives is provided in the Auditory Skills Curriculum manual. Sample activities are included for each of the IPOs. All activities should be designed to facilitate the achievement of objectives with the age of the student in mind. The trainers are encouraged to add variations as well as new activities.

The Audio Worksheets are designed for use with the curriculum and the TAC. They provide assessment and training materials for all objectives except for those in the area of auditory feedback. The artwork and auditory stimuli have been field tested and revised.

The TAC is a widely used clinical and educational tool in this country. The additional curriculum materials provide a valuable guide for auditory skills training, particularly for advocates of a multisensory approach. The IPOs and activities reflect the Sanders (1982) philosophy of following a sequence beginning with highly redundant situations and progressing to decreasingly redundant situations. There is also focus on holistic perception or "chunking" where the listener does not deal with word-by-word input but, rather, "chunks" of information from phrases to paragraphs, within which many more perceptual clues are embedded than are found in words alone.

LISTENING SKILLS PROGRAM

In Utah, both the auditory-oral (AO) approach and the total communication (TC) approaches are available options through the statewide Utah School for the Deaf (USD), which serves children and youth with moderate to total bilateral hearing loss. Previously, the parent-infant auditory program of the USD was described. With or without parent-infant training, children often enter the USD at age 3 years. Emphasis is placed on providing a continuation of auditory training under what is called the Listening Skills Program (LSP). The LSP has been strongly influenced by Dan Ling, Leahea Grammatico, and Doreen Pollack. Audiologists and teachers of the hearing-impaired collaborate in providing LSP students with binaural amplification and listening, speech, and language training. Focus is placed on the development of natural language and normal speech and early integration with normal hearing peers. The unisensory auditory approach is used rather than a multisensory approach. Lipreading is not encouraged.

Individual tutoring in listening and speech is given to young USD children daily. The Ling Five Sound Test and other methods are used to check hearing aids and earmolds every day. The listening and speech targets of the tutoring sessions are included in classroom and home learning experiences. The TAC, the Ling Phonetic Speech Evaluation, and the Grammatical Analysis of Elicited Language (GAEL) scales are administered yearly or more often. Videotapes of listening and speech performance of each child are made twice a year.

A tutoring session for a child may last 20 minutes. Individual goals are written and individualized materials developed. Children are trained to listen and speak following the Ling program, to repeat vocal music lines, and to remember and repeat increasing numbers of words associated with pictures from individual notebooks. Children learn to recognize animal sounds, to tell stories from picture referents, to answer questions about stories and to ask questions, to converse about interesting happenings, and to sing with appropriate melody. The data demonstrate that the LSP is a generally effective approach for development of listening skills. The USD staff state that children in this program have dramatically increased both speech and listening competency. The results of the LSP at the USD have been so encouraging that the school is seeking legislative funds to increase staff so that all hearing-impaired students of the school who can benefit may receive listening and speech tutoring and follow-up school and home verbal communicative assistance.

AUDITORY-VERBAL COMMUNICATION

The term "auditory-verbal" is used now instead of "auditory oral" by many members of the Alexander Graham Bell Association for the Deaf (AGBAD). A special group of the AGBAD has been set up and is called the International Committee on Auditory-Verbal Communication (ICAVC). This committee hopes to ensure that "each child with a hearing impairment has the opportunity to acquire natural auditory verbal communication at an early age. Members of the ICAVC seek to accomplish this goal through information dissemination, demonstrations, collaborative research, special training, providing discussion forums, identifying successful programs, and advocating education in the regular schools whenever possible. The ICAVC advocates the development of auditory-verbal communication for severely and profoundly hearing-impaired children through:

1. Promoting early detection programs;
2. The earliest possible use of the most appropriate form of amplification for the child, usually binaural;
3. Teaching the child to acquire and process language through the habitual and maximal use of residual hearing regardless of auditory acuity;
4. Expecting the child to function independently in the most normal learning and living environment;

5. One-to-one teaching;
6. A parent/caretaker-centered approach;
7. The development of auditory self-monitoring of speech;
8. The development of spoken language communication—that is, living and learning through natural sound spoken language communication; and,
9. Diagnosis and prognosis in the course of ongoing evaluative therapy.

LISTENING REFINEMENT PROGRAM

Once a hearing-impaired child has developed a basic foundation in listening, language, and speech, the need exists to refine the child's communication skills. A speech refinement program developed by Berg and Child (1985) has previously been described in this chapter. Now a listening refinement program (LRP) concurrently developed by Berg and Child (in press), and its correlation with speech refinement, will be outlined.

Listening and speech are reciprocally related and mutually supportive. Listening refers to the detection, discrimination, recognition, and comprehension of speech, primarily, and nonspeech or environmental stimuli secondarily. Speech refers to voice, prosody, and the articulation of vowels and consonants. During listening training, speech perception is emphasized but speech production is also given attention. When voice, prosody, or articulation training is emphasized, listening to speech is required also.

Listening to speech requires auditory (A), visual (V) and/or AV speech perception. Listening performance may be measured by percentage of words, sentences, or messages understood. In the LRP, a unique listening test is administered. This test provides up to 9 subtests which involve combinations of 3 sensory conditions (A, V, and AV) and 3 levels of speech (words, sentences, and messages). The test is not standardized, but is useful. It can be administered in 15 minutes.

Table 6-5 summarizes the A, V, and AV scores of one hard-of-hearing college student on the Berg listening test. Generally, this student performed better visually than auditorily. As expected, he also generally scored higher under the AV condition than he did under either the A or V condition. He varied widely in comprehending messages under the 3 sensory conditions.

These scores give a rough initial estimate of the overall listening performance of this student under 9 conditions. Further testing and diagnostic training are recommended to clarify these findings. Tentatively, it appears that this student is a phenomenal lipreader and does not need visual listening training. The student also appears to be competent auditorily except when trying to comprehend messages through audition.

The listening refinement program includes 5 levels of speech discrimination, recognition, or comprehension training: (1) prosodic discrimination;

Table 6-5.
Percentage scores of hard-of-hearing students under auditory,
visual, and auditory-visual listening conditions using words,
sentences, and messages

Listening Measure	Auditory	Visual	Auditory-Visual
Phonemes in CVC words	73	97	90
Words in sentences	92	90	98
Concepts in messages	38	63	87

(2) sentence recognition; (3) word recognition; (4) phonetic discrimination;
and, (5) message comprehension. To administer auditory training in the case
described above, only the phonetic discrimination and message comprehension tasks of the program are recommended. For clients with lower listening
baselines, lower level tasks would be administered initially until pass or fail
criteria were met.

The LRP provides up to 163 discrimination, recognition, or comprehension tasks. Each discrimination task includes 3–5 closed-set items. Each
recognition task typically includes 10 open-set items. Each comprehension
task includes a message from 2 to 7 sentences in length. Pictures are included
with the discrimination task items. The level of tasks and particular tasks
included in listening training are selected for each individual student based
on test scores and other relevant information. An example of each of the 5
levels or types of tasks are given below.

1. Prosodic discrimination: (*chair, table, bicycle, television*)
2. Phonetic discrimination: (*beet, bit, bait, bet, bat*)
3. Word recognition: (*swim, stun, fret, bikes, etc.*)
4. Sentence recognition: (*Write your last name on the paper, etc.*)
5. Message comprehension: (*A red fox lives in the meadow near the
   woods. It hunts for food at night. It eats meadow mice. It likes to steal
   chickens.*)

A hearing-impaired student progresses through the tasks selected for
training as fast as possible. Procedures and criteria have been arbitrarily
written. Feedback is given and progress assessed often enough to keep the
client motivated and learning. If a student is not progressing with one task,
another, more appropriate, task is used. The task can be given under A, V,
and AV conditions. Discrimination and recognition tasks are completed before the messages are administered. Ordinarily, these tasks are presented
unisensorily. The messages are also given unisensorily if discrimination and
recognition pass criteria have been met unisensorily. If not, the messages are
given under the AV condition. Ordinarily, training is conducted in a quiet
environment. Afterwards, competing noise can be introduced if desired. The
A, V, and AV test and training data on a student are useful in predicting
listening success in a classroom.

SELF INSTRUCTION

To reach full capacity in listening and speech, the child or youth needs extensive practice. Normally, this practice is provided through incidental daily learning experiences provided by the environment and with no special effort required of a child. Children with normal hearing accurately recognize the salient characteristics of both their own speech and that of others and usually find listening and speaking highly useful and rewarding. If a child has a hearing loss, that child often needs special stimulation and training to learn to listen and speak, and then needs additional practice to solidify or habituate spoken communicative skills. Special assistance is also needed to re-establish listening and speech skills when they have been neglected after being learned in the first place. Self-training is an economical way to provide at least some of the listening and speech practice needed by the hearing-impaired student.

Self-instructional tasks give the student the opportunity to practice a listening skill or speech target that is introduced initially through "live" interaction. Self-instruction should probably be delayed until the child is in elementary school and has developed considerable basic communicative competence. Someone familiar with the tasks involved in self-instruction should be in the student's vicinity periodically to give instructions, answer questions, and prompt learning.

The Listening Refinement Programs have been converted to self-instructional tasks. The instructions for learning the discrimination and recognition tasks differ from those of learning messages. With a discrimination or recognition program, each task or list contains sublists which are randomizations of the original list. A student is instructed to listen to each sublist item, write it down on a script, move a cover card to reveal the correct answer, and write down the number of correct responses at the end of each sublist. If the student does not meet the pass criterion after going through all the sublists, that student can repeat the sublists or discontinue the task.

Each message task requires that a student listen to the entire message and then write down answers to questions about that message. After answering all questions for that message and checking for accuracy, the student writes down the number of correct responses. Each task is presented only once, except that the student reviews it if any responses to questions are incorrect. The student then proceeds to the next task or message. Four levels of messages are included, each longer than the previous level. A student has to respond correctly to 2 consecutive messages (pass criterion) to advance to a succeeding level (Berg, Blair, Ivory, Viehweg, Watkins, 1983).

The Audio Worksheets of the ASIPS also provide assessment and practice materials for objectives in areas of auditory discrimination, memory sequencing, and figure ground. Eighty-six tasks require the student to mark responses on self-check worksheets. The majority of tasks use pictures and the remaining tasks a simple printed vocabulary. The cassettes are recorded with a 150-

Hz stop pulse between items, for use with a program-stop recorder. The ASIPS also includes a manual entitled "Media for Auditory Training," which includes a description of the program-stop recorder, the widely used Bell & Howell Language Master card reader, and a school center where students can come for listening activities.

Self-instructional speech practice ordinarily makes use of an electrovisual indicating device like the Vocal Scope. The student is given a list of words or sentences containing a target phoneme that the student can say correctly. The student practices the use of the target phoneme in these additional speech contexts. A person initially assists the hearing-impaired student to recognize the radial pattern of the target phoneme. The word and sentence stimuli of the 133 SRP articulation programs are particularly useful for self-instruction.

Hearing-impaired students can also practice voice, prosody, and oral-nasal targets by themselves. Simple and more complex targets can be practiced with electrovisual devices. A hard-of-hearing student may have hypernasality in addition to misarticulations. The TONAR (the oral nasal acoustic ratio) computerized device has been developed by Fletcher (1972) to measure and modify nasality during continuous utterance. The student speaks into a sound separator microphone assembly. Panel lights indicate progress toward criteria. Currently no instrument provides a comparative automatic indication of speech articulation accuracy. The Visi-Pitch and Sound Spectrographic displays, like the Vocal Scope, do not automatically indicate voice or speech accuracy but do provide helpful visual patterns that correspond to various speech and voice parameters. Electrovisual voice and speech aids may become widely accepted in speech clinics.

STUDY PROGRAMS FOR PARENTS AND TEACHERS

An indispensable facet of a listening or speech program for a hearing-impaired child is the understanding and participation of parents and teachers. Both parents and teachers should be involved and supportive. In instances in which specialists are not involved, parents and teachers potentially have an even larger role to fulfill if the child's communicative needs are to be met. Currently, parents and many teachers are largely uninformed with respect to how to assist with listening and speech training, except for parents of infants and of preschoolers. Knowledgeable and supportive parents and teachers make the difference between hearing-impaired children learning to listen and speak effectively or not.

A new national service for parents and teachers of the hearing impaired has recently been established (Berg, 1985). Parents or teachers may subscribe to a weekly newsletter and educational audiology course that focus on listening and speech skills. A basic 40-week course is provided as well as additional services and products. Videotape demonstrations will accompany illustrated, printed materials. The course does not require prerequisite coursework but covers the content of an extensive educational audiology course. University credit may be received for completion of assignments and examinations. Workshops provide hands-on experience with equipment and materials. Individual assistance is provided by Berg or arranged through referral to educational audiologists who live close to the subscribers. Arrangements for visits to exemplary programs are facilitated and purchase information on equipment and materials provided.

In the basic 40-week course, each lesson includes 2 topics with related practicum. For example, the first lesson describes the "listening area" and "listening and speech development". A total of 80 topics are covered. Parents and teachers learn not only what they can do but what educational audiologists and other school personnel need to do to improve listening, speech, and related abilities. Other topics include *sound, the ear, hearing, audiograms, tympanograms, hearing and speech aids, room acoustics, room amplification equipment, the telephone,* and the Individualized Educational Program (IEP).

Another project of Berg, (1984) is designed to educate prospective career educators in providing classroom listening support in the elementary and secondary schools, especially to hard-of-hearing children and youth. The project is entitled Listening in Urban and Rural Noise (LURN), to emphasize the need to alter the typically poor acoustical and listening conditions in school classrooms. Project LURN will be implemented in many universities during 1985–1988.

The latter project for prospective teachers will be centered around a competency-based course called Listening for the Hard-of-Hearing Child. Seven course modules will be included: (1) hearing considerations; (2) relevance of audiograms; (3) personal hearing aids; their operation and maintenance; (4) sound in classrooms; (5) listening and speech skills; (6) frequency modulation equipment; and, (7) IEPs. The listening course will be offered through preservice delivery to university students majoring in elementary, secondary, and special education, and to university personnel who supervise student teaching. Instructional materials will include a handbook, video demonstrations, and microcomputer disks. The listening course will be taught during successive academic-year quarters by educational audiologists. Instruction will be offered through class and individual study and competencies applied during student teaching experience.

SUMMARY

It seems obvious that listening and speech skills are attainable by the great majority of hearing-impaired students in regular and special schools. The programs described in this chapter provide vehicles for planning and implementing appropriate strategies for improving listening and speech. Other chapters also contain applicable information. More than 30 years ago, Erik Wedenberg (1954) stated that the goal of auditory training was that a hearing-impaired student score normally on a test of verbal intelligence. The relevance of listening and speech training to this goal remains.

REFERENCES

Auditory skills instructional planning system. Los Angeles County Schools. North Hollywood: Foreworks.

Berg F. Language development. In F Berg & S Fletcher (Eds.), *The hard of hearing child.* New York: Grune & Stratton, 1970, 111–124.

Berg F. *Educational audiology: Hearing and speech management.* New York: Grune & Stratton, 1976.

Berg F. *Listening in urban and rural noise.* Proposal submitted to Handicapped Personnnel Preparation, Office of Special Education, U. S. Department of Education, Washington, D.C., November 9, 1984.

Berg F. *Home study program in educational audiology.* Smithfield, Utah: EAR Products and Services, 1985.

Berg F, Blair J, Frantz J, Ivory R, Viehweg S, & Watkins S. *Listening in classrooms, hard of hearing.* Final report, Regional Education Programs for Deaf and Other Handicapped Persons (Postsecondary), Office of Special Education, U. S. Office of Education, Washington, D.C., July 1983.

Berg F & Child D. Precision listening and speech programs. Orlando: Grune & Stratton, (in press).

Bokelmann D. *Training aides to administer transfer programs and discrimination booklet.* Las Vegas: Clarke County School District, 1973.

Boothroyd A. *Hearing Impairments in young children.* Englewood Cliffs, N.J.: Prentice-Hall, 1982.

Clark T & Watkins S. *Programming for hearing impaired infants through amplification and home intervention.* Logan, Utah: Utah State University, 1985.

Erber N. *Auditory training.* Washington, D.C.: Alexander Graham Bell Association for the Deaf, 1982.

Fletcher S. Tonar II: An instrument for use in management of nasality. *Alabama Journal of Medical Science,* 1972, *9,* 333–338.

Geers A, Moog J, & Schick B. Acquisition of spoken and signed English by profoundly deaf children. *Journal of Speech and Hearing Disorders,* 1984, *4,* 378–388.

Horton K. Every child should be given a chance to benefit from acoustic input. *Volta Review,* 1973, *75,* 348–350.

The International Committee on Auditory-Verbal communication means "deaf" children learning to hear and speak naturally. Pamphlet. Washington, D.C.: Alexander Graham Bell Association of the Deaf.

Ling D. *Speech and the hearing impaired child.* Washington, D.C.: Alexander Graham Bell Association for the Deaf, 1976.

Ling D. *Cumulative record of speech skill acquisition.* Washington, D.C.: Alexander Graham Bell Association for the Deaf, 1978a.

Ling D. *Teacher/clincian's planbook and guide to the development of speech skills.* Washington, D.C.: Alexander Graham Bell Association for the Deaf, 1978b.

Ling D. The detection factor (videotape). Montreal: McGill University, 1981.

Lundsteen S. *Listening : Its impact on reading and the other language arts.* Urbana, Ill.: National Council of Teachers of English Educational Resources Information Center, 1971.

Magner M. *Speech intelligibility test for deaf children.* Northampton, Mass.: Clarke School for the Deaf, 1972.

McLean J. *Shifting stimulus control of articulation responses by operant techniques,* Demonstration project report No. 82. Lawrence, Kan.: Parsons Research Center, 1967.

Nicholls G, & Ling D. Cued speech and the reception of spoken language. *Journal of Speech and Hearing Research,* 1982, *25*(2), 262–269.

Pollack D. *Educational audiology for the infant and pre-schooler.* Springfield, Ill.: Charles Thomas, 1985.

Prescott R, & Turz M. *Auditory pattern recognition by young hearing impaired children.* Wahington, D.C.: Federal City College, 1975.

Ross M. *Hard of hearing children in regular schools.* Englewood Cliffs, N. J.: Prentice-Hall, 1982, 3–7.

Sanders D. *Aural rehabilitation: A management model.* Englewood Cliffs. N. J.: Prentice-Hall, 1982, 374–379.

Subtelney J, Orlando M & Whitehead R. *Speech and voice characteristics of the deaf.* Washington, D.C.: Alexander Graham Bell Association for the Deaf, 1981.

Watkins S. *Longitudinal study of the effects of home intervention on hearing impaired children.* Unpublished doctoral dissertation, Utah State University, 1984.

Wedenberg E. Auditory training of severly hard of hearing preschool children. *Acta Otolaryngologica.* Supplementum 54, 1–129.

Wedenberg E, & Wedenberg M. The advantages of auditory training: A case report. In F Berg & S Fletcher (Eds.) *The hard of hearing child.* New York: Grune & Stratton, 1970, pp. 319–330.

Frederick S. Berg

7

Classroom Acoustics and Signal Transmission

This chapter addresses the related topics of classroom acoustics, transmission, and amplification. The hearing-impaired child in school may experience a variety of acoustical and stimulus presentation conditions. Understanding the nature of sound, its propagation, the signal-to-noise ratio (S/N), reverberation time, and compensatory signal transmission and classroom amplification technologies provides a basis for assisting the child to listen more effectively in school.

THE FACETS OF SOUND

Sound may be defined as vibration which can be heard through a propagated change in the density of an elastic medium such as air. When a person speaks, or when sound is produced in some other way, sound waves travel from the sound source to many different locations multidirectionally. Direct and reflected vibrational change reaches listeners who are within earshot. The ear is particularly sensitive and responsive to vibrational energy between 250 Hertz (Hz) and 4000 Hz, although vibration rates between 16 Hz and 23,000 Hz may be heard by some people. Direct and reflected sound ordinarily reaches the listener within a fraction of a second after it originates. Sound waves travel through air at a speed of about one-fifth of a mile each second (1130 ft/sec).

All sound sources except for tuning forks or electronically produced tones vibrate at many frequencies simultaneously. Each vowel or musical tone is made up of harmonically related frequencies. Voiceless consonants or other noise-like sounds include a great many randomly produced frequencies. Both

157

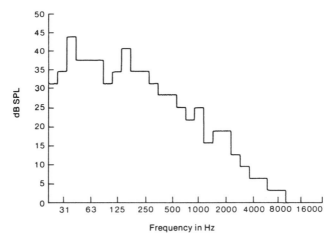

Fig. 7-1. Noise floor plat of unoccupied classroom.

harmonically and inharmonically composed sounds can be broken down into a fixed number of single-frequency sounds or pure tones, each with a particular amplitude depending on the sound. A pure tone vibrates sinusoidally about a point of reference. On an oscilloscope, this sinusoidal change is seen as a sine wave. On the same instrument, other sounds which are composed of two or more sine waves are seen as complex waves.

The school environment is filled with various sounds from myriad sources. Some sounds are desirable and are called "signals". Other sounds are undesirable and are called "noise". The teacher's voice, for example, is the signal and competing voices or other sounds, the noise. Usually there are more noises than signals. Even at night, when a classroom is unoccupied and supposedly quiet, there is background noise present. This noise is referred to as the noise floor. Figure 7-1 shows a typical noise floor of a classroom at night. The noise levels are greatest for the low frequencies and become progressively less at higher and higher frequencies. During the day, and particularly when occupied, the noise floor increases in overall intensity and in high-frequency composition because of the inclusion of human voices, particularly children's voices.

The vertical scale of Figure 7-1 reads in decibels (dB) which are derived from logarithmic values based on powers of 10. The highest intensity level of any sound frequency of the noise floor is 44 dB, or 6.435 x 10 x 10 x 10 x 10 (64,350) times as intense as 0 dB, or absolute hearing threshold for a 1000-Hz tone. The overall decibel level of all sound frequencies of this noise floor is shown as 53 dB. If the intensity level in decibels of all frequencies present were figured cummulatively, they would equal 53 dB, or sound 724,300 times as intense as a 1000-Hz sound at 0 dB.

The data below provide sound intensity references for conceptualizing overall decibel values. Whereas the room above was 53 dB, the values below vary from 0 to 100 dB.

dB	Ratio	Condition
0	1:1	Normal hearing threshold at ear
20	100:1	Soft whisper at 1 meter
40	10,000:1	Quiet room
60	1,000,000:1	Quiet conversation at 1 meter
80	100,000,000:1	Very noisy classroom
100	10,000,000,000:1	Shout at 1 meter

Three speech signal values—soft whisper, quiet conversation, and shout—are specified above at one meter distance. The decibel levels of these signals differ at different distances; the intensity level of the noise, however, might be more constant throughout a room, due to reverberation.

In an unbounded space, sound becomes less and less intense proportionate to the square of the distance from the sound source. Doubling the distance decreases sound intensity to one fourth its previous value or by 6 dB; and tripling the distance decreases intensity to one ninth or by 9.54 dB. The overall intensity level of quiet conversation from a distance of one meter averages approximately 60 dB. Accordingly, at 2 meters it would be 54 dB, at 4 meters 48 dB, and at 8 meters (about 25 feet) 42 dB. In a bounded space, such as a classroom, sound level does not decrease as much as in an unbounded space with increasing distance because both reflected and direct sound are present.

The signal is the sound we desire to hear and the noise the sound that is interfering with what we want to hear. The intensity of the signal should be considerably greater than the intensity of the noise so that listening will be effective. The signal-to-noise ratio is of critical importance to the listener. A S/N ratio of 0 dB means that both the signal and noise have the same intensity. A S/N ratio of +10 means that the signal is 10 dB more intense than the noise. A S/N ratio of -10 dB means that the noise is 10 dB more intense than the signal. In the classroom with the 53-dB overall noise level, the listener at one meter from a talker would hear soft conversation (60 dB) at a +7 dB S/N ratio. At 2 meters and then 4 meters, the S/N ratio would decrease accordingly, making listening more and more difficult. These distance differences are not as noticeable when lipreading is possible in addition to using hearing for listening.

When a person puts on a hearing aid, both the signal level and the noise level are heard more intensely. The S/N *ratio* stays where it was without sound amplification. If the S/N ratio was undesirable without an aid, it is still undesirable with the aid. Noise is a deterrent to listening. It is essential to locate noise sources and reduce their dB levels. Noise or an inadequate S/N ratio not only deleteriously effects listening but hearing measurement at low signal levels. This is why a booth isolated from extraneous noise is needed for absolute threshold hearing measurement.

Another listening deterrent is too much reflected sound or reverberation. This causes noise to build up in intensity and the signal to smear in the temporal domain. The floor of noise that exists in a room has already been discussed. Reverberation, however, refers more particularly to excessive repeated reflection of the speech signal. While reflection adds to direct transmission to make a speech sound more intense, it also masks the direct speech sound. Rather than a word appearing sound-by-sound, the sounds become superimposed on successive sounds, smearing them. The greater the reverberation, the greater the speech smearing.

Reverberation time (RT) is the time required for a sound that is produced to reduce 60 dB in intensity once that sound has been shut off. The absorption coefficients of the surfaces of the room and, to a much lesser extent, the volume of the room, determine the reverberation time. If these coefficients are very low, which happens when surfaces are hard and nonporous, a sound will reverberate a great deal. If these coefficients are very high, a sound will be absorbed into the surfaces and direct, nonsmeared sound will predominate.

Reverberation times vary from near 0 seconds in an anechoic room to several seconds in a reverberant chamber. The anechoic room does not allow sound to reflect. The reverberant chamber does not allow sound to be absorbed quickly. An organ is usually placed in a hard-surfaced room to permit its sounds to reverberate. In this same room, talkers will find it hard for their listeners to understand them.

A schematic of direct sound, early reflections, and closely packed reverberant sound is shown in Figure 7-2. If there is no reflected sound, a room will sound dead. A normal listener appreciates at least some reflection, but a hard-of-hearing person listens more effectively if only direct sound is present, provided that sound is made intense enough to be heard comfortably.

Consonant sounds are particularly smeared or masked because they are relatively weak and short in duration and thus more susceptible to closely packed reverberant reflection than are nonconsonant sounds. Consonants are also smeared more because they include relatively more high-frequency energy, which room surfaces generally absorb well. The place features of consonants, which depend greatly upon high-frequency cues for correct perception, are particularly adversely affected by room reverberation. The combination of room reverberation and excessive noise accelerates the deterioration of listening performance.

Sound is also affected by the location and isolation of a room. The further

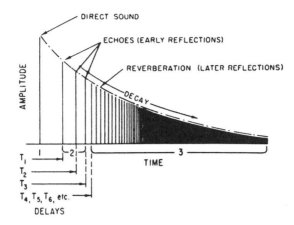

Fig. 7-2. Schematic of direct sound, early reflections, and closely packed reverberant sound. (From Woram).

the room is from external noise, the better. Also, the more the room is built to keep outside noises from getting in, the better. A school that is located in a quiet neighborhood and has sound-isolated rooms is ideal. If considerable outside noise is present, room isolation is that much more important. External noise will pass through walls unless they contain materials that will dissipate sound by converting the sound energy to heat. Cracks in doors and other openings also provide paths for incoming noises. These sounds enter as reflections or diffractions of transmitted waves.

CLASSROOM LISTENING DATA

The classroom noise level and reverberation time influence substantially the degree to which students can understand the teacher. The typical school classroom has an occupied noise level of 60 dB or more and a reverberation time of more than 0.4 seconds, both of which are undesirable for hard-of-hearing students (Ross, 1978).

Obviously, the listening effectiveness of hard-of-hearing students is more disrupted by excessive noise or reverberation than is that of normal hearing students. The effects are illustrated in Table 7-1, which presents speech discrimination scores of school-age children under several noise and reverberation conditions. Listening scores are compared at 0.4- and 1.2-second RTs and with S/N ratios of 0, +6, and +12 dB. The normal hearing students had mean scores of 95 percent and the hard-of-hearing students had mean scores

Table 7-1.
Average speech discrimination scores of 12 normal hearing
students and 12 hard-of-hearing students under RTs and
S/N ratios simulating various classroom conditions

RTs (in seconds)	S/N Ratios (in dB)	Percentage of Words Repeated	
		Normal	H-of-H
0.4	+12	83	60
	+6	71	52
	0	48	28
1.2	+12	70	41
	+6	54	27
	0	30	11

From Finitzo-Hieber T & Tillman T. Room acoustics' effects on monosyllabic word discrimination ability for normal and hearing impaired children. *Journal of Speech and Hearing Research,* 1978, *21,* 440–458. With permission.

of 83 percent when tested in an audiometric booth with little or no reverberation and noise.

The 0.4- and 1.2-second RTs represent classrooms which are acoustically
treated and not acoustically treated, respectively. The + 12 dB S/N ratio has
been considered minimally acceptable for a hard-of-hearing student in a
classroom. The + 6 and 0 dB S/N ratios are fairly typical of school classrooms.
The scores of Table 7-1 indicate that even normal hearing students cannot
listen optimally in a typically noisy school classroom, even when the room is
acoustically treated (0.4 second RT).

The "hard-of-hearing" data in Table 7-1 are for students with bilateral
hearing loss. It is likely that the listening scores of students with unilateral
hearing loss would fall somewhere between the scores of normal hearing
students and those of students with bilateral hearing loss. In a recent laboratory study, Bess (1982) found that students with unilateral hearing loss
experience learning difficulties in classrooms, even when given preferential
seating (teacher facing normal ear of student).

NOISE AND REVERBERATION MEASUREMENT

Instruments are available for measurement and evaluation of sound
pressure levels and reverberation times. Sound pressure in dynes/cm² can
be converted to sound intensity in watts/cm² because intensity is proportional
to the square of the pressure. The sound level meter reads in decibels Sound
Pressure Level (SPL) re: 0.0002 dynes/cm² or Intensity Level (IL) re:

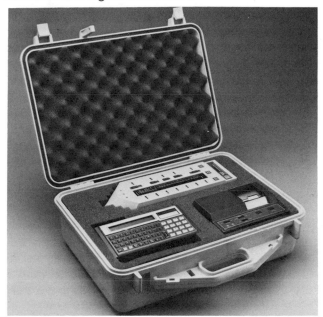

Fig. 7-3. Larson-Davis 800B Precision Sound Level Meter in carryng case with computer, printer, and mass memory drive unit. Compliments Larson-Davis.

.0000000000000001 watts/cm², which equates to both the pressure (SPL) and intensity units (IL). Use of the sound level meter is commonplace in educational audiology, whereas use of reverberation analysis equipment is not.

The Larson-Davis Laboratories provide state-of-the-art equipment for making many types of measurements at reasonable cost. Figure 7-3 shows a complete battery-operated system for programming, taking, and printing measurements. This fully portable system can automatically measure: (1) sound levels from -10 dB to 140 dB at octave or one third octave intervals from one Hz to 20,000 Hz; and, (2) RTs at various frequencies. A companion portable dosimeter/sound level meter permits samples of overall sound measures in decibels to be obtained over periods as long as 2 weeks. The data can be dumped and printed out at any time.

A less expensive but more limited sound level meter can be used to get overall signal or noise measurements at specific times. Quest Electronics manufactures a small, portable meter with a series of lights, each corresponding to 2-dB steps above 50 dB. Any sound with a pressure or intensity between 50 and 90 dB will cause a light to go on, or a series of lights in order of varying decibel levels.

An Apple IIe computer program has been written to estimate, rather than measure, RT. It is based on the formula:

$$RT = \frac{0.05\,V}{A}$$

RT is measured in seconds, V (volume) of the room in cubic feet, and A (total absorption) in sabins. The total absorption is the sum of the separate absorption of the 4 walls, ceiling, and floor of a room. The absorption of each of these 6 areas is the product of the average absorption coefficient and the area in square feet. The average absorption coefficient is the mean of coefficients at 500, 1000, and 2000 Hz. The absorption coefficients at a series of frequencies for each of a number of common surface materials are shown in Table 7-2.

The RT computer program provides an estimated RT quite rapidly. The information entered is: (1) length, width, and height of room; and, (2) length, width, and surface material of each of the 6 areas. After entering data from a number of rooms and seeing the estimated RTs, one can almost estimate RTs without taking measurements or entering data into the computer program. Generally, the RT for a small room with a rug on the floor and acoustic tile on the ceiling is going to be less than 0.5 seconds. If a rug is not present, the RT may be 0.7 seconds. If both the rug and ceiling tile are absent, the RT may be over one second. Ordinarily, the walls of rooms are not treated and are hard and nonporous. Drapes further reduce reverberation time, as do soft objects and people in a room. The actual RT, however, is best obtained by using special equipment. Estimated RTs often may be within 0.1 second of measured RTs.

REDUCING NOISE AND REVERBERATION

Each school classroom should be as free of noise and reverberation as possible to enhance effective listening. Noise is generated outside schools and within schools and is generated outside classrooms, and within classrooms. Reverberation results from hard, nonporous, or inelastic materials with which both noise and signal come in contact.

Noise Reduction

Ideally, a school should not be built in a locality in which there is a high level of noise. If it is, the school should be isolated from excessive noise by partitions or other surfaces which reflect or absorb sound. In the school itself, excessively intense sounds should either not be generated, or, if generated,

Table 7-2.

Absorption coefficients for various materials (including people)

Material	125 Hz	250 Hz	500 Hz	1000 Hz	2000 Hz	5000 Hz
Marble or glazed tile	.01	.01	.01	.01	.02	.02
Concrete, unpainted, smooth	.01	.01	.01	.02	.02	.03
Brick, unglazed	.03	.03	.03	.04	.05	.07
Carpet, heavy on concrete	.05	.10	.30	.50	.60	.65
Carpet, heavy on felt over concrete	.08	.25	.60	.70	.72	.75
Carpet indoor-outdoor over concrete	.01	.05	.10	.20	.40	.60
Concrete, painted	.10	.05	.06	.07	.09	.08
Concrete, unpainted, coarse	.36	.44	.30	.30	.40	.25
Linoleum or tile on concrete	.02	.03	.03	.03	.03	.02
Wood floor	.15	.11	.10	.07	.06	.07
Wood over concrete	.04	.04	.07	.06	.06	.07
Acoustical tile, ceiling	.8	.9	.9	.95	.9	.85
Curtains, light velour	.03	.04	.10	.20	.25	.35
Curtains, medium velour	.07	.30	.50	.75	.70	.60
Curtains, heavy velour	.15	.35	.55	.75	.70	.65
Glass, ordinary window	.35	.25	.20	.10	.07	.04
Glass, heavy plate	.18	.06	.04	.03	.02	.02
Plasterboard on wood studs	.30	.15	.10	.05	.04	.03
Plywood paneling on studs	.30	.20	.15	.10	.09	.09
Plaster on concrete or brick	.10	.10	.08	.05	.05	.05
Fiberglass 3 cm thick	.2	.5	.9	.95	.9	.85
Water surface as in swimming pool	.01	.01	.01	.02	.02	.03
Audience, absorption per person in sabins	0.35	0.43	0.47	0.50	0.55	0.60

should be isolated from classrooms and other places where teachers and students are located. In classrooms, noisy equipment should not be allowed; teachers' and students' voices should be kept low; and rugs and acoustic tile should be used to dissipate sound.

Noise studies of schools and classrooms reveal that much needs to be done to improve the acoustical environments in which students learn. This chapter will refer to some of these studies in which overall noise in schools and classrooms has been measured with sound level meters set at A, B, and C weightings. These weightings correspond to the 40-, 70-, and 100-phon contours for normal hearing. The 40-phon curve is the equal loudness contour that has a loudness of one sone, equivalent to soft conversational speech. The 70-phon curve has a loudness of 12 sones, equivalent to moderately loud conversational speech. The 100-phon curve has a loudness of 85 sones, reflecting an intensely loud sound. Each phon curve is plotted by connecting intensity points from low to high audible frequencies which sound equally loud. Because the 40 (A), 70 (B), and 100 (C) phon curves (weightings) increasingly give as much emphasis to low-frequency sound as to mid- and high-frequency sound, for the same overall sound being measured, the A weighting reads lowest in decibels, the B weighting somewhat higher in decibels, and the C weighting highest in decibels.

Finitzo-Hieber (1981) recently presented noise measurement data on a variety of representative school classrooms in the Dallas and Chicago areas. The data Finitzo-Hieber presented on decibel (A) measures in occupied rooms are summarized below.

1. The traditional classroom with 25 students and one teacher had a noise level of about 60 db.
2. The open-plan classroom with 100 students and 10 teachers had a noise level above 70 dB.
3. The mainstream classroom for hearing-impaired students had about as much noise as the traditional classroom.
4. A carpeted classroom in a school for the hearing impaired with 5 students and one teacher had a noise level from 40–45 dB.
5. Gymnasiums, cafeterias, and terminal rooms had decibel noise levels between 70 and 90.

Generally, the noise picture of these schools was bleak. The exception was the school for the hearing impaired, where provision had been made to reduce occupied classroom noise to almost the same level as unoccupied classroom noise.

The noise levels presented by Finitzo-Hieber (1981) are in general agreement with those found by other investigators. Ross and Giolas (1971) found the ambient room noise to be 60 dB (C) in a classroom selected to be average in size, location, and acoustics. Sanders (1965) found mean decibel (B) noise values of kindergarten classes to be 69, high school 62, elementary 59, and units for the hearing impaired 52.

In a study of fairly modern classrooms used by elementary and junior high hearing-impaired students, Sinclair, Riggs, Bess, and Lang (1980) found that the median decibel (A,B,C) unoccupied noise levels were 41, 50, and 58 (respectively). The corresponding occupied noise levels were 56, 60, and 63 (respectively). The 15-dB increase in the A scale reading was a result of additional high-frequency noise contributed by the students. It is of interest that all these classrooms had acoustic ceiling tiles, most had carpeting, and

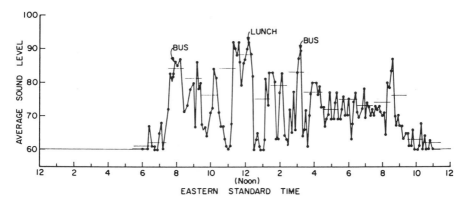

Fig. 7-4. Dosimeter measures during a school day of a 13-year old boy.

approximately half had acoustic wall tiles across at least a portion of the wall surface.

Johnson (1979) studied the sound exposure his 13 year old son received from the time he got up one morning to late that evening. Figure 7-4 shows a breakdown of dosimeter measurements taken every 3 minutes. The horizontal bars are hourly averages. The sound intensity levels exceeded 60 dB (A) the great majority of the time and 90 dB (A) at times. Note particularly the intense decibel (A) levels encountered by his son on the school bus or when he was eating lunch. In a rowdy science class, the levels exceeded 80 dB. Only when one of the teachers was strict with a class were the sound readings in the low 60s. The particular meter being used was not designed to read below 60 dB (A). The decibel (A) readings were from signals and noises produced by the boy and other persons and by noise from sources in and out of school. The meter was worn continually.

Bess & McConnell (1981) suggest minimum overall noise (dB—A) level criteria for classrooms for the hearing impaired. These criteria are 45 dB (A) in classrooms where children learn special skills such as arts and crafts or physical education, but still use hearing aids, and 30 or 35 dB (A) in classrooms where children spend the greatest amount of time and in which effective use of hearing aids is most important for learning.

Minimum noise level criteria for specific frequency regions have also been recommended. These values are derived from octave measurements from 31.5 Hz through 8000 Hz. When an octave band analysis is made, the data can then be plotted on a Noise Criteria (NC) curve. This curve is compared with a family of NC curves to determine its relative value. The members of the family of NC curves are given values. An NC 30 curve corresponds to an overall noise level of 35 dB (A). The lower the NC level, the better the listening condition. Gengel (1971) stated that when speech is delivered to a hearing aid at a level of about 60 dB SPL at a distance between 3 and 15 feet (as in conversational speech), the ambient noise level should not exceed 30 dB (A), or about NC 20–25. The corresponding minimum noise levels for normal hearing students are 35 dB (A) and NC 30.

The discrepancy between recommended and actual noise levels in school classrooms varies from 25 dB (A) for traditional classrooms to 30–35 dB (A) for open-plan classrooms. Further studies need to be conducted to determine the extent to which a series of decibel (A) noise levels interfere with listening effectiveness of students in schools. Gengel (1971) stated that a + 12-dB S/N ratio was minimally acceptable for hearing-impaired listeners. Berg, Blair, Frantz, Ivory, Viehweg, & Watkins (1983) discovered that one group of hard-of-hearing college students listened effectively with hearing aids in an acoustically treated room having an ambient noise level of 53 dB (A) and S/N ratio of + 12 dB. The teacher's speech signal was at 65 dB (A).

One is tempted to recommend a practical minimum noise level of 50 dB (A) or below for a classroom. Hard-of-hearing students vary, however, in their ability to tolerate competing noise when they are tyring to listen to speech. Speech intelligibility data obtained in a test booth for 9 hard-of-hearing college students exemplifies individual effects of recorded speech babble. The mean drop in speech intelligibility with competing babble at 0 dB S/N ratio was 10.8 percent. Individuals ranged from a 4-percent drop to a 26-percent drop (Berg et al., 1983). A minimum acceptable noise level for each student needs to be determined.

Study also needs to be made of the effect upon overall noise of eliminating or reducing each outside or inside noise. A sample of outside and inside noises contributing to overall decibel-level and listening problems is listed below. A noise list for each school and each classroom in a school should be generated. Attention should be given to eliminating, reducing, or isolating each noise source.

1. Sonic boom from jet aircraft
2. Incessant rumble or vehicular traffic
3. Horseplay of exuberant youngsters in hall
4. Vibration from ventilators, heaters, and projectors
5. Machine noises from workshops and crafts rooms
6. Unnecessary talk, foot shuffling, and paper crumpling

Special attention should be given to keeping noise from entering classrooms and to reducing noise within classrooms. Solid-core doors, double-paned windows, heavy construction walls with air spaces, carpeting, and acoustic tile are all helpful. A quiet room provides an improved learning and teaching environment for all concerned.

Open-space classrooms should be eliminated or spaces within them acoustically isolated from one another. Currently, their S/N ratios are negative or completely acoustically unacceptable, even for normal hearing students. The acoustical disadvantage outweighs the sum of all the advantages of these

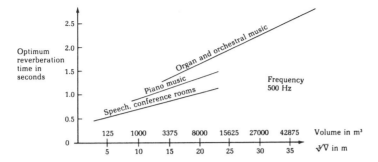

Fig. 7-5. Optimum speech room RTs for normal hearing students.

spaces. Major school funds need to be allocated for reconstruction of these spaces within schools. The open-space classroom has proven as much an educational disaster as asbestos insulation has proven a health disaster.

Reverberation Reduction

The Finitzo-Hieber & Tillman (1978) data presented earlier suggest the need to reduce RT in school classrooms. What acoustical engineers consider optimum speech room RTs for normal hearing students are shown in Figure 7-5. If 2 rooms have the same acoustical treatment, but one is larger than the other, the optimum RT for the second increases by a ratio of about 1/20. Optimum RTs for hard-of-hearing persons are lower than for normal individuals. Nabalek (1976) suggests that hard-of-hearing students might listen most effectively if the RT is reduced to O.

A practical goal for a school classroom of typical size, about 10 meters long by 6 meters wide by 2.5 meters high, might be to maintain a RT of no longer than 0.3 seconds. This might be achieved if the ceiling has acoustical tile and the floor has carpet with padding. These surface materials, plus the teacher and students, might provide sufficient sound absorption for effective listening. In constructing new schools, acoustical tile is typically used as well as carpet to a considerable extent. Familiarity with the RT formula and with average absorption coefficients of surface materials and people provides a basis for making fairly accurate estimates of room RT. Even clapping hands and listening for reverberation is a useful technique.

A joint program of reverberation reduction and noise reduction in classrooms and other learning stations of a school is a highly desirable educational goal. The reduction of RT is easier to achieve, however, than is the reduction of noise. In classrooms, halls, gymnasiums, cafeterias, and shops, noise seems to abound just because exuberant students are present. Perhaps the education establishment can take a lesson from the business establishment, where there is increasing recognition that poor acoustics are annoying and hamper worker efficiency.

Commercial Materials

There are commercially available materials that are particularly effective for reducing noise and reverberation. The SONEX absorptive sheets of the Illbruck Corporation of Minneapolis are made of foam in "anechoic wedge" shapes. Noise striking the foam is converted into noiseless heat energy. The wedges serve to further dissipate the noise by the process of deflection. These sheets present a surface area up to 450 percent greater than that of a flat material of the same dimensions.

SONEX-type materials can be attached to walls, ceilings, room or desk partitions, or can be hung as baffles. They are positioned to absorb sound by its source. The 1985 cost is $39.50 for a box of four 2-feet by 2-feet sheets, or about $2.50/square foot. The sheets can be trimmed to fit various areas. Owens Corning Corporation produces fiberglass panels with comparable high-absorption coefficients for less than $1 a square foot. These panels are designed for ceilings but can be adapted for wall or partition use.

In planning the acoustics of a room, 2 types of noise control are considered: (1) the Noise Reduction Coefficient (NRC) rating, an average of the absorption coefficients of the material for the frequencies 250, 500, 1000, and 2000 Hz; and, (2) the Sound Transmission Class (STC) value, a measure of the ability of a wall to resist sound passage. The STC value is particularly important when a classroom is adjacent to high noise levels. Mineral fiberboard may have a 35–40 STC value, which effectively keeps computer room and cafeteria noise out of classrooms. The mineral fiber substrate also provides a tackable surface that may be used as a bulletin board and to hold lightweight pictures. All materials used should be fire-resistant.

SIGNAL TRANSMISSION AND AMPLIFICATION

In lieu of, or in addition to, noise and reverberation reduction, sound transmission and amplification technologies help children listen more effectively in school. The transmission technologies include frequency modulation (FM), electromagnetic, and infrared equipment. The amplification technologies include electronic amplifiers and electroacoustic transducers. These technologies provide a way for the speech signal to effectively bypass room noise and reverberation. The improved signal level applies to any person activating a transmitter. At school, that person ordinarily is the classroom teacher, whereas at home it is one of the parents. In theory, any number of persons could activate signal transmitters.

In school, sound transmission equipment has a distinct advantage over infrared transmission equipment. This advantage lies in the multidirectionality of radio waves and unidirectionality of infrared waves. The sound transmitter the teacher or parent is wearing does not have to be facing the listener, whereas the infrared transmitter does. Also, if sunlight enters a room in which infrared transmission is used, it interferes with signal transmission. Infrared transmission is effective, however, in auditoriums and if a teacher always faces the students in a classroom. Infrared transmission is also effective in TV rooms.

Personal FM

The personal FM system is the most commonly employed transmission-amplification technology used with hearing-impaired children. This system includes an FM receiver and the personal hearing aid worn by the child. At the signal end of the system, the teacher or parent may wear a wireless lapel microphone, transmitter, and antenna. A speech signal is transduced into an equivalent electrical signal, which modulates and is carried on a transmitted radio wave to a radio receiver worn by the child. The antenna of the radio receiver picks up the transmitted signal which in turn, is demodulated in the radio receiver worn by the child. The signal is then delivered through direct wire or through electromagnetic induction to the child's hearing aid. Theoretically, the original signal arrives at the listener's ear as if the speaker were inches away rather than many feet away. The resulting S/N ratio may meet optimal acoustical criteria for school classrooms.

An FM system includes a wireless microphone transmitter worn by a talker and radio receiver worn by a listener. Both the FM transmitting unit and receiving unit from one major company weighs 4 ounces. There are omni-directional, unidirectional, or noise-cancelling micropone options for transmitting in quiet to noisy to very noisy environments. Plug-in channels selector crystals permit narrow-band FM transmission. Wide-band FM transmission is also available. The transmitter or receiver may fit into a pocket or into a pouch clipped on a belt. Nine-volt batteries are used, either rechargeable nickel-cadmium or alkaline. A nicad battery charger may be used. Figure 7-6 shows the components of this system.

Some FM companies build the radio receiver to function also as a hearing aid. A switch on such a unit permits environmental sound and/or FM signal input. A less expensive and perhaps better option is to interface the FM receiver with the listener's personal hearing aid. A switch on the hearing aid can permit environmental and/or FM signal input. In this way, a hearing aid selected for the listener's hearing loss can be used.

Three options are available for interfacing an FM receiver to a personal hearing aid. One is direct electrical wire connection from the receiver to the hearing aid. A second is direct electrical wire connection to a transducer attached to the outside of a hearing aid. With this option, the electrical signal is transduced into a sound signal and fed into the hearing aid microphone. A third option is delivering the electrical signal to a wire loop placed around the neck of the listener. With this option, the magnetic field of the loop induces

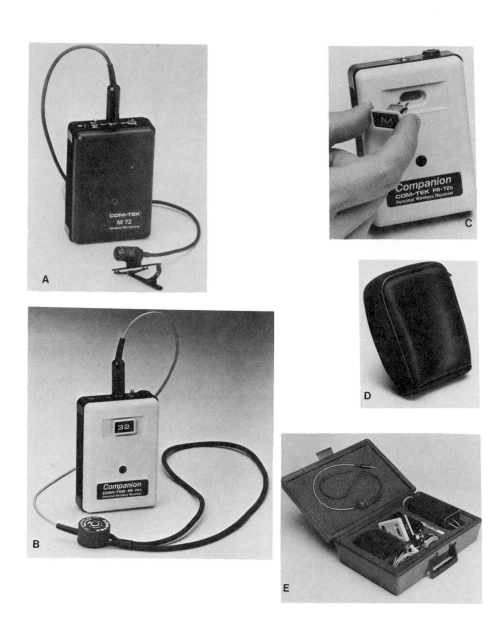

Fig. 7-6. Components of an FM system designed to be interfaced with a personal hearing aid. Compliments Communications Technology.

an electrical signal in the telephone coil of a hearing aid. The electrical and inductive options are both commonly used. The acoustic transducer option has not gathered support, perhaps because environmental sound as well as transduced sound is free to enter the hearing aid microphone. Often, the environmental sound is noise background.

Inductive coupling was the only input option when FM systems were first interfaced with personal hearing aids. Van Tassell and Landin (1980) described this as the personal inductance loop or FM mini-loop, which was worn around the student's neck. The receiver signal was routed to this loop and signal transduction accomplished by the telecoil in the student's personal ear-level aid(s). The signal was then amplified and delivered to the student's hearing aid receiver and earmold. Since classroom induction loops had previously provided gross variations in signal strength, Van Tassell and Landin hypothesized that the audiologist might expect similar signal irregularities with the FM mini-loop.

Van Tassell and Landin then compared the frequency responses of 5 hearing aids when using microphone input versus FM mini-loop interface. The results showed that the audiologist could not predict the latter from the former frequency responses. For example, one aid that provided a high-frequency response with the microphone no longer did when interfaced with the FM mini-loop. Van Tassell and Landin also compared clinic and classroom conventional FM sensitivity. Clinic measures were taken through the environmental microphone of the FM unit used as a hearing aid. Classroom measures were taken with FM units approximately 20 feet from the teacher microphone-transmitter-antenna. The frequency responses were similar, but the gain across frequency in the classroom was reduced an average of 18 dB from what it was in the clinic. Van Tassell and Landin's experiments suggest that indiscriminate use of FM equipment in classrooms is not justified and points to the need to evaluate all FM systems before they are used.

Direct electrical wire input into hearing aids has increased in popularity since the Van Tassell and Landin study. Many power ear-level aids now include electrical inputs. Not only severely and profoundly hearing-impaired listeners may need personal FM aids, however, but also children with less severe hearing impairment.

Berg et al. (1983) also compared several signal transmission and amplification options. Their subjects were college students with bilateral hearing loss from 25 to 65 dB. These students had previously been subjected to lengthy hearing tests, hearing aid evaluations, and listening training. They were fitted with hearing aids that provided them with comparatively good amplification. Aided speech recognition scores were individually obtained initially in audiometric test booths under quiet and 0-dB S/N conditions. Aided speech recognition scores were also obtained through group testing in an old classroom with a 1.67-second RT, with and without 12 dB of public address amplification. Table 7-3 details the individual listening scores achieved by each of the 9 subjects.

Table 7-3.
Hearing Loss as measured in listening percentages of 9 hard of hearing subjects under 2 test booth and 2 classroom conditions

Environmental Conditions	Hard-of-Hearing Subjects and Hearing Loss in dB										
	1	2	3	4	5	6	7	8	9	Mean	SD
	55	20	30	40	65	35	65	60	65	48	
Audiometric test booth with hearing aid in quiet	84	98	90	82	86	92	80	92	88	88.00	5.66
Audiometric test booth with hearing aid in noise	80	84	52	64	58	45	78	20	86	63.00	21.81
Highly reverberant room with hearing aid	28	78	32	12	26	76	22	22	30	36.22	23.84
Highly reverberant room with hearing aid and public address system	50	90	28	24	26	94	36	40	44	48.00	26.00

The listening scores obtained with hearing aids in quiet in the audiometric test booths were the standards against which listening scores under all other conditions could be compared. The mean standard was 88 percent. Each subject achieved a listening standard of at least 80 percent in the test booth. The standard deviation among subjects for this condition was 5.66 percent, which is comparatively small. The mean listening percentages for these same subjects under the other 3 conditions varied from 63.00 to 36.22 to 48. The individual variations for these other conditions were great. Corresponding standard deviations were 21.8–26 percent.

Additional listening scores of these subjects were obtained using many different FM options. In some instances, FM brands (Com Tek, Earmark, Phonic Ear, and Telex) were compared. In other instances, FM coupling arrangements were varied. Comparisons were also made between room RTs (1.67, 0.69, and 0.47 seconds). The FM equipment was used as it came from the manufacturers. Great listening percentage variations occurred. For example, the listening score of one subject using an FM receiver as a hearing aid in the 1.67-second RT room was only 11 percent. In the same room, however, the mean percentage of subjects using one brand of FM with inductive (loop) coupling was 84.88. The loop scores were generally as high as listening scores in quiet in test booths, except for the scores of 2 subjects whose percentages were 56 and 60 percent. Fewer subjects used two other FM brands in the 1.67-second RT room, listening only half as effectively with electrical or acoustical (transducer) coupling to their hearing aids.

In the 0.47-second RT room, subjects listened effectively using hearing aid, public address amplification, personalized FM with inductive (loop) coupling, and FM receivers electrically coupled to button receivers attached to earmolds. Mean scores of 5–7 of the 9 subjects under these conditions were

75, 80, 77.5, and 80 percent, respectively. The similarity of these scores suggests that FM equipment may not be critical for a room that is fairly quiet (53 dB overall and relatively non-reverberant).

In the 0.69-second RT room, listening scores of two of the subjects were compared under hearing aid conditions and while using the two most popular personalized FM input options, electrical and loop. All four FM brands were involved in these comparisons. Mean listening percentages varied from 4 (personal FM electrical) to 85 (personal FM loop). The mean score of another personal FM electrical option, however, was 84 percent.

Nault (1983) studied factors related to FM mini-loop coupling to personal hearing aids. Noise output, frequency response, and listening data on 5 hard-of-hearing college students were compared. Listening data included test booth measures of word recognition and classroom measures of sentence recognition. The reverberation time of the classroom was 0.69 seconds. Monaural and binaural hearing aids, 3 FM mini-loop arrangements, and a combined FM receiver and hearing aid electrically connected to a button receiver were used. Environmental microphone and FM reception options were employed with the FM system connected to the button receiver.

Findings from Nault's study were that: (1) The mini-loop consistently introduced noise; (2) The hearing aid outputs were reduced when coupled to the FM mini-loops in two of three instances; (3) The effects of increased noise and reduced outputs did not significantly affect classroom listening scores; (4) Listening with one of the FM mini-loops in the classroom was effective and, (5) Listening with the FM system coupled electrically to the button receiver was effective. The latter 2 FM systems increased the subjects' speech listening scores by 37 percent as compared to scores while using hearing aids alone. These classroom averages were almost as high as the audiometric test booth scores. When the other 2 FM systems were coupled to hearing aids through mini-loops, however, the classroom listening scores were depressed.

In support of the Van Tassell and Landin study cited above, the direct wire system resulted in an advantageous S/N ratio. Nault's subjects reported, however, that they would not wear this system, whereas they would use the mini-loop system because it was hidden, and, therefore, more cosmetically appealing. Since the Nault data and previously cited Berg et al. (1983) data revealed that an FM mini-loop can result in listening scores comparable to test booth scores with hearing aids under quiet conditions, and since telecoils are more common in personal hearing aids than are electrical inputs, the FM mini-loop system should continue to be commercially available.

Hawkins (1984) recently compared several hearing aid arrangements and a number of personal FM combinations in a 0.6-second RT classroom using 9 children with mild to moderate hearing loss. The listening scores of the subjects did not differ with electrical versus inductive (mini-loop) FM couplings to hearing aids. Hawkins noted that the advantage of personal FM over hearing aids alone is equivalent to an improvement of 12–18 dB in S/N, even when children have favorable classroom seating. He also found that: (1) The magnitude of the personal FM advantage decreases as the classroom S/N improves; (2) There is still a personal FM advantage when the child is seated close to the teacher; and, (3) The advantage of FM systems with environmental microphones is reduced substantially when their environmental microphones are activated. Hawkins also noted that the preferred classroom hearing aid arrangement was binaural amplification with directional microphones.

Sound-Field FM

The FM signal can also be transmitted to a common FM receiver-amplifier coupled to electroacoustic speakers. The talker with the transmitter is mobile, but all students now hear a transmitted-amplified signal. Such a sound-field FM system can result in a S/N at listeners' ears of + 12 dB. The person with the microphone transmitter can speak with no more than moderate effort and be heard well, provided the classroom noise level is kept below 60–65 dB (A). Two speakers are recommended, either attached to tiles that are substituted for removable ceiling tiles or installed in room corners. Sound-field FM equipment has just recently been made available commercially at a cost of approximately $1500, including installation costs, as indicated in Figure 7-7. Like personal FM equipment, sound field FM equipment should be evaluated to determine S/N and listening effectiveness.

Ideally, each schoolchild, with or without hearing loss, should have the advantage of a very positive S/N ratio. Even normal hearing children miss important speech signals when teachers are at a distance, and particularly when they turn their faces away from students. The option to a transmitted-amplified signal is for the teacher to raise her voice or move closer to children. If another student is the talker to be heard, this child often is not heard well enough to hold the attention of other students in the class. Recorded music

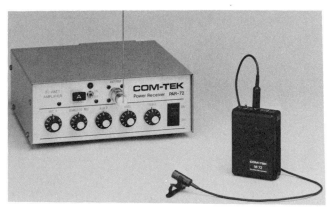

Fig. 7-7. A sound field FM system. Compliments Communications Technology.

can also be similarly transmitted and amplified to students while they are doing independent study in a classroom, resulting in significantly less distractions due to competing noise.

Sarff (1981) described the benefits of sound-field FM equipment with 4th-, 5th-, and 6th-grade students with minimal hearing loss and the equipment's associated academic benefits. The effectiveness of sound-field FM treatment in overcoming academic deficits was compared to the effectiveness of resource classroom treatment. Both treatments were effective, but the FM treatment was the more effective. Other advantages of FM were that: (1) Hearing-impaired children did not have to be singled out; (2) Normal hearing children benefitted also; and, (3) Cost/classroom was $1500, purchase price, as compared to $15,000/year for a resource teacher. In addition, teachers generally preferred the equipment because they did not have to overexert their voices. Sarff cautioned, however, against using sound field equipment in extremely noisy classrooms or in situations where the signal would have to be amplified to be greater than 75 dB Hearing Level (HL). He recommended other sound treatment procedures prior to installation of sound-field FM equipment.

Recently, Jones (1985) studied the effectiveness of sound-field FM equipment in kindergarten classrooms of a school district in which he serves as the educational audiologist. Three acoustically similar kindergarten classrooms were selected, each with unoccupied noise levels from 51 to 55 dB and RTs between 0.3 and 0.4 seconds. Thirty-six subjects were selected from 6 classes (6 subjects from each class) of 5- and 6-year old children who used the 3 kindergarten classrooms. Each subject had sufficient receptive vocabulary to comprehend NU-Chips (Elliot & Katz, 1980) listening test items.

The 6 kindergarten children from each class included 3 hard-of-hearing (experimental) subjects and 3 normal hearing (control) subjects. These children were selected from 25-30 students in the class, just prior to the experiment to be described. Impedance and pure-tone screening tests were administered to each child in a mobile test booth. The experimental subjects were selected from among those children with middle ear pathology and minimal hearing loss according to screening results. The control subjects were selected randomly from children who did not have ear or hearing problems according to screening results.

The subjects from each class were seated at 3 desks in the center of a classroom. Each of the hard-of-hearing and normal hearing subjects marked multiple-choice pictures in response to test words from a tape recorder under 3 different treatments. In the first treatment (A), the tape recorder was placed on a teacher's desk in one corner of the classroom and no amplification was provided. The second treatment (B) was identical, except that the recorder was placed on a desk close to the center of the classroom. The third treatment (C) was identical to treatment A, except that the signal was delivered to 2 ceiling tile speakers through sound-field FM transmission and amplification. Treatment A was described as distance listening without amplification. Treatment B was described as close listening without amplification. Treatment C was described as distance listening with amplification. The S/N ratios under treatments A, B, and C were approximately 0 dB, +6 dB, and +12 dB, respectively.

The mean listening percentages of the 18 hard-of-hearing subjects under treatments A, B, and C were 81.3, 96.0, and 97.8, respectively. The comparative percentages for the 18 normal hearing subjects were 91.2, 98.4, and 98.4, respectively for treatments A, B, and C. The groups (experimental and control) and the results for first treatment versus other treatments were significantly different. Since the NU-Chips Listening Test is easy compared to most kindergarten listening tasks and since the room acoustics were comparatively good, the results of the Jones study suggest that: (1) A serious listening problem exists in kindergarten classes when a teacher is at a distance from hard-of-hearing students; and, (2) This listening problem may be alleviated either by a teacher moving close to communicate with students or by using sound-field FM equipment. The former solution should be used as often as possible until appropriate sound-field devices can be installed.

Cost Savings Options

An alternative to use of electroacoustic speakers in a sound-field FM classroom arrangement is use of an inductance loop. The FM signal is still picked up by a common FM receiver-amplifier, but it is then electrically fed into a loop of wire. The electrical signal is accompanied by a surrounding magnetic signal that induces corresponding electrical signals in the telecoils of students' hearing aids. The signal strength across the room may be most constant, without spilling over to adjacent rooms, if several small loops in series or parallel or in series/parallel combinations, are installed under a thick rug on the floor.

An audio-induction loop system permits hearing-impaired children with hearing aid telephone coils to listen successfully to FM radio, to a motion picture sound track, to a teacher using wireless FM transmission, to stereo (with normal hearing children simultaneously listening through speakers), to TV, to a car radio, and to a radio or cassette recorder while jogging (Smith, 1985). If a wireless microphone-transmitter is not available, a microphone can be wired to a miniature microphone located at the teacher's desk.

The teacher can communicate with the entire class by replacing the inductance loop with electroacoustic speakers. The S/N ratio for this system might be +12 dB, and for the inductance loop and hearing aid telecoil arrangement +24 dB. The electroacoustic speaker arrangement might be practical for students with normal hearing or minimal hearing loss who do not use personal hearing aids. In comparison with the sound-field FM system, a wired microphone would however, *only* allow the teacher to reach the students with improved S/N ratios when at the teacher's desk, unless the teacher is willing to use an extended-length wire. High-quality components for a nonradio-transmission system can be purchased at RadioShack or other electronic supply houses for $200–500. The alternative to electronic room systems is for the teacher to talk at close range to students or to raise the voice when speaking from a distance.

There is a potentially huge market for signal transmission and classroom amplification technologies. Up to now, that market has been largely restricted to students with severe and profound hearing loss. In the future, the market will, it is to be hoped, extend to students with less severe hearing impairments and even to the normally hearing population of students in the nation's schools.

SUMMARY

There are formidable room acoustic problems in the homes and schools of the nation. These problems are largely unrecognized or misunderstood. Excessive noise and reverberation is commonplace, deleteriously affecting the listening and learning of all students, particularly those with hearing loss. Steps can be taken to reduce acoustical problems to manageable proportions. Acoustical modifications can be made. In addition, signal transmission and amplification equipment can be installed in classrooms.

REFERENCES

Berg F, Blair J, Frantz J, Ivory R, Viehweg S, & Watkins S. *Listening in classrooms, hard of hearing,* Final report, Regional Education Programs for Deaf and Other Handicapped Persons (Postsecondary), Grant No. G008101357, U.S. Department of Education. Logan, Utah: Utah State University, July 1983.

Bess F. Children with unilateral hearing loss. *Journal of the Academy of Rehabilitative Audiology.* 1982, *15,* 131–144.

Bess F. & McConnell F. *Audiology, education, & the hearing impaired child.* St. Louis: C.V. Mosby, 1981.

Elliot L & Katz D. Northwestern University Children's Perception of Speech (NU-CHIPS). St. Louis, Auditec, 1980.

Finitzo-Hieber, T. Classroom acoustics. In R Roeser & M Downs (Eds.), *Auditory disorders in school children.* New York: Thieme-Stratton, 1981, pp. 250–262.

Finitzo-Hieber T & Tillman T. Room acoustics' effects on monosyllabic word discrimination ability for normal and hearing impaired children. *Journal of Speech and Hearing Research,* 1978, *21,* 440–458.

Gengel R. Acceptable speech-to-noise ratios for aided speech discrimination of the hearing impaired. *Journal of Auditory Research,* 1971, *11,* 219–221.

Hawkins D. Comparisons of speech recognition in noise by mildly-to-moderately hearing-impaired children using hearing aids and FM systems. *Journal of Speech and Hearing Disorders.* 1984, *49,* 409–418.

Johnson D. *Why Is The Noise Dose of Humans Important.* Unpublished presentation, Dayton, Ohio: Wright-Patterson Air Force Base, Aerospace Medical Research Laboratory, 1979.

Jones J. *Listening of kindergarten students under close, distant, and sound field FM amplification conditions.* Unpublished educational specialists thesis, Utah State University, (in press).

Nabelek A. Reverberation effects for normal and hearing impaired listeners. In S Hirsh D Eldrege, I Hirsh, & SR Silverman (Eds.), *Hearing and Davis,* St. Louis: Washington University Press, 1976, pp. 333–341.

Nault D. *The effects of selected electroacoustic properties of FM systems on speech discrimination of moderately hearing impaired individuals in a reverberant classroom condition.* Unpublished masters thesis, Utah State University, 1983.

Ross M. Classroom acoustics and speech intelligibility. In J Katz (Ed.), *Handbook of clinical audiology.* Baltimore: Williams & Walkins, 1978, pp. 469–478.

Ross M & Giolas T. Three classroom listening conditions on speech intelligibility. *American Annals of the Deaf,* 1971, *116,* 580–584.

Sanders D. Noise conditions in normal school classrooms. *Exceptional Children,* 1965, *31,* 344–353.

Sarff L. An innovative use of free field amplification in regular classrooms. In R Roeser & M Downs (Eds.), *Auditory disorders in school children.* New York: Thieme-Stratton, 1981, pp. 263–272.

Sinclair J, Riggs D, Bess F, & Lang S. *Classroom noise in schools for the hearing impaired.* Paper presented to the Tennessee Speech and Hearing Association, Nashville, Tennessee, April 1980.

Smith C. Induction loop systems. *Hearing Instruments.* 1985, *36,* 26; 31.

Van Tassell D & Landin D. Frequency response characteristic of FM mini-loop auditory trainers. *Journal of Speech and Hearing Disorders,* 1980, *45,* 247–258.

Ann L. Wilson-Vlotman

8

Management and Coordination of Services to the Hard of Hearing Child

One of the strongest single forces in operation in American education today is the drive to guarantee the rights of the handicapped. It has resulted in a succession of federal laws which have provided many opportunities for children who are handicapped and which have prohibited discrimination against handicapped persons in any federally aided program. It has also resulted in a strong move to mainstream as many children as possible through the "least restrictive placement" clause of Public Law 94-142 (U.S. House of Representatives, 1975. In addition, the "related services" component of this law has provided a way to meet the unique needs of handicapped children in a mainstream setting. Audiology is one of these related services to be provided for children with hearing handicaps.

The focus of this chapter is on the changing roles of parents, teachers, and administrators in meeting the needs of the hard-of-hearing child in the regular classroom and on the responsibilities of the educational audiologist in the process of change.

Chapter 2 elaborated upon the current status of educational audiology as examined by Wilson-Vlotman (1984). It was discovered in this national study that educational audiologists are continuing to provide a clinic-based service to the school population. They were found to be providing minimal consultative services to school personnel, and almost no direct service (tutoring speech, language development, listening training) to students. It was felt that educational audiologists had little understanding about, or skill in, implementing change in public schools, and that they were meeting unprec-

181

edented problems in their job situations (Wilson-Vlotman, 1984). The issue of initiating change in public schools is considered at length in this chapter and is examined in terms of the problems and needs of educational audiologists who are trying to effectively impact classrooms.

IMPLEMENTING CHANGE IN SCHOOLS

Modern organizations, of which the school is one, need to cope with many internal and external attempts at change; however, historically many organizations are very slow to change. Schools are no exception.

Basically, change is directed at altering the behavior of those in the organization. This is not an easy task due to the fact that it is very threatening to the security of the individuals. Administrators may see attempts at change as a challenge to their organization, for which they may have great feeling of ownership. Educational audiologists would do well to understand how change works to enable them to commence the process of making audiology in the schools an essential and complete service to students and staff, while bringing the school to full compliance with the law.

To be effective, change must be initiated by the educational audiologist and the school administration as the result of sound planning. Several principles should be kept in mind when a change in attitudes of administrators, teachers and parents is planned.

(1) *A planned, systematic program must be initiated by the school's management.* Long-term change must have the approval of the power sources, the decision-makers. Educational audiologists can begin to effect change by working with individual teachers and parents in eliciting support for improving the audiological service, but ultimately the change will need to be approved by administrators. Change involves a great expenditure of social, emotional, political, and economic resources both within and without the school.

(2) *The program must aim at making the organization more adaptable to either the present or the anticipated environment.* Change requires much planning. Schools are quite inflexible in their operations and seemingly changeless, but effective change has been successfully implemented where those in the organization believe in it. Administrators must be made aware of the current status of the program, be encouraged to ask questions, seek opinions, and see the potential benefits of preparing for change.When change does occur, those involved must have a personal commitment to it and must be willing to adapt accordingly, of their own free will. Change will result in a modification of teacher behavior patterns, which must be tolerated by the administration. The adaptation necessary is no where better highlighted than in the need to facilitate the mainstreaming so popular during the last decade. Effective classroom/teacher change means teachers must have practical

activities that fit their situations, or be shown through actual demonstration accompanied by personal support. Then they become more adaptable to change.

(3) *The program must use methods designed to change knowledge, skills, attitudes, processes, behaviors, and job and organizational design.* Effective change affects all dimensions of the organization and the individual. Teachers must find out about hearing loss, they must believe they can contribute to the betterment of the hearing-impaired child's learning potential. Added resources of equipment, space, and time are needed for added projects. Personal involvement in acquiring knowledge of and planning the implementation of the program, and personal recognition for involvement must occur for each planned change. Educational audiologists should always remember to start where the lay person is, and not where they themselves are in knowledge of the field, whenever initiating change. People not techniques make change.

Educational audiologists must realize that they are personally instrumental in creating a need for recognition of their program. They are also responsible for carrying through much of the planning for teacher change. Implementing change is a complex process, "participation, continued support and resources, and the excitement of becoming competent are all part of the needed conditions for improvement" (Lieberman & Miller, 1984, p. 94).

IMPLEMENTING CHANGE IN AUDIOLOGICAL PRACTICES IN SCHOOLS

Lewin (1947) drew attention to what he viewed as the 3 stages of change. First, "unfreezing" is the stimulation of people to feeling and recognizing change. People are threatened by new ideas, and when confronted with different ways of looking at what they do, whether it be teachers being told that what they have done is inadequate, or educational audiologists being faced with the need to do more than diagnostics and assessment. Educational audiologists might ask themselves why so many of their number, even though they are working in schools, remain in the clinical mode of operation and are failing to deal with the educational implications of identified hearing loss in children. Are they threatened by the refocus of audiology when training has not prepared them to deal with it? Preparation for leadership roles is noticeably absent from audiology training programs, adding to the audiologist's overall inability to cope with change.

Those who call for change, who are challenged by it, and who have identified need areas are at the second stage of change, which involves participating in new ways of doing things. The "refreezing", or third stage, involves seeing that new ideas, skills and knowledge are part of the system.

Szilagyi and Wallace (1980) refer to a level of tension which is antecedent to any successful change. School administrators may feel pressure to decide whether or not the move is wise, while teachers may be genuinely concerned about added responsibilities. The educational audiologist must give the confidence necessary to redirect that tension, and must build self-esteem in the teachers and other school personnel responsible for working with the child who is hearing impaired. All this takes time to initiate, time which must be spent in becoming known, listening to others, offering help and taking opportunities to speak at meetings where influential people are gathered. Confidence in the service planned will follow confidence in the person proposing the changes.

There is no doubt that implementing change is challenging. Identifying those with power who will support the change is mandatory. Principals are important, and may even be critical to effective change, but they are not the only initiators of change. Principals without ideas can be, and are, led by others. School secretaries have been known to wield enormous power, as have secondary administrators. Locate these persons and work with them, for it is their opinion which will weigh the most in any decisions regarding change.

School personnel are extremely concerned about the impact on students of any innovation. Mainstreaming was forced upon many schools and became a practice without an administrative advocate for a vast number of handicapped children who entered the public school system. Educational audiologists have a role to play for which no one has currently taken responsibility. Who is presently managing the needs of hard-of-hearing children in schools? Teachers of the deaf are trained to be concerned with academics and speech-language pathologists maintain a too-large direct service caseload and have not indicated a feeling of responsibility for hearing aid management. Persons skilled in auditory management are needed. They must go beyond assessment of the child to a full-service provision of consultation, indirect service, and perhaps some direct service (Wilson-Vlotman, 1984). It may be that these persons do not provide all needed services, but they must see to it that services are provided.

One way the problems of inadequate service to hard-of-hearing students can be handled is to change the way these students are treated in the regular schools. As suggested earlier, too often a clinical model of treatment is used. The child is taken out of the classroom by any one of a number of specialists and is provided with individual or group therapy for 20–60 minutes, 2–5 times each week. The only way this type of treatment can truly benefit the child is when the activities in the session outside the classroom are coordinated with teachers activities and synchronized with the activities going on in the child's homeroom (Ross, 1979).

An alternative way to treat children is to provide the individual services needed by the child as part of the ongoing learning in the regular classroom. Perhaps the educational audiologist can work with a small group of children, one of them the hard-of-hearing child, in the areas of language and reading within the classroom itself, following the general lesson plans and objectives of the teacher. The child will benefit from the specialist, but will also benefit from the continuity of being in the classroom and being exposed to activities and experiences of the other children. While assisting the child, the educational audiologist is also developing a trusting relationship with the teacher, who has possibly never known what happens when a child leaves the room for special attention. The educational audiologist begins, ideally, to develop an advocacy relationship for the services offered to the teacher.

If the above suggestions are to be implemented, educational audiologists will need to spend more quality time with regular classroom teachers than is now the case. According to Wilson-Vlotman (1984), educational audiologists spend, on the average 1–2 hours a month consulting with classroom teachers. Yet, educational audiologists sampled felt that these teachers have only moderate skill in working with hearing-impaired children. There is thus a critical need for quality input to regular teachers if services are to be improved. This input must come from someone who respects and appreciates the regular classroom teacher. The educational audiologist and the teacher need to be able to talk together as colleagues. There must be a reciprocal relationship built on trust and respect so that the educational audiologist can both teach and learn in this kind of relationship, and thus initiate changes in service provisions. The primary objective in the relationship, however, is to help the teacher to change, to be able to provide more of what the hearing-impaired child needs.

SUPPORTING AND TRAINING TEACHERS

Over the years, regular classroom teachers who have taught hearing-impaired students have felt a great deal of isolation, frustration, and helplessness in dealing with the child who is struggling to keep up with the remainder of the class, and who often has social problems.

Mainstreaming has become a popular concept, and much has been written of the troubles and prospects facing the child who is mainstreamed. Many hearing-impaired children have failed to meet expectations of this placement and blame has been thrown in numerous directions. Misconceptions concerning mainstreaming are common:

1. Physical placement alone in the regular school is often viewed as being the criterion for success.
2. Regular classroom teachers who may have no knowledge and sometimes little interest are expected to meet all the needs of the hearing-impaired child along with those of all other children at a time when administrative paperwork has become overwhelming.

3. Itinerant teachers of the deaf are sometimes expected to provide all the support needed in the classroom.
4. Itinerant teachers of the deaf are assumed to have the necessary training to work in mainstream settings when, in actual fact, very few have these skills.
5. There is no perceived need for a special coordinator of services to main-streamed, hearing-impaired children and families, nor a perceived need for trained administrators.

These misconceptions continue to exist, and a result of poor planning is seen in the failure of regular classroom placement to provide more than any segregated placement is able to achieve. Mainstreaming has captured the imagination but not come to terms with many issues. While overall educational goals are the same for all children, methods to achieve these goals vary. The indiscriminate, uncoordinated placement of a hearing-impaired child in the mainstream is unjust to all concerned. The child becomes the innocent recipient of inadequate services. Parents generally do not know specifically what their child needs; administrators are not fully aware of the ramifications of a hearing loss and of their legal responsibilities to the child. The regular classroom teacher is trapped, for usual teaching methods aren't always appropriate. The educational audiologist can become the mainstream case manager and coordinate the delivery of services to the child. It is suggested that the challenge of working with hearing-impaired children in the mainstream can be very rewarding if teachers are supported appropriately. Those who have experienced the challenge will testify to the fact that being a classroom teacher of normal children is time-consuming. To add to the classroom a handicapped child with unique needs adds another dimension. More intense, personalized planning is required for a handicapped child than for a normal child, along with a comprehensive knowledge of some of the educational implications of that handicap. Additional meetings and paperwork are involved in a mainstreaming programs and many interruptions are added to the school day by support personnel, all demanding full attention. While these are not insurmountable problems, they do exist and must be dealt with. A child's success in the mainstream classroom is dependent upon the regular classroom teacher being fully supported. Haphazard coordination of the classroom placement does not ensure the least restrictive placement for a child with special needs.

Needs of the Regular Classroom Teacher

What do regular classroom teachers need from an educational audiologist in order to function effectively and how could these needs be met? The following suggestions for developing a successful audiological program should be viewed alongside the Model of Delivery of Service as described in Chapter 2 and Figure 8-1.

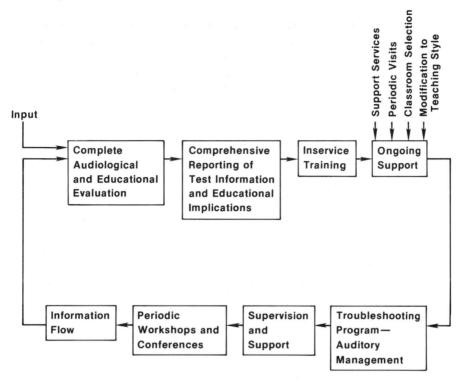

Fig. 8-1. The cycle of responsibility of educational audiologists to classroom teachers.

The flow chart in Figure 8-2 describes the cycle of responsibility of educational audiologists to the classroom teachers with whom they work. At the input level, the child is referred to the school audiological service and the process of identification and diagnosis begins. Educational audiologists are subsequently responsible for more than many have seen as their role responsibility, including:

1. *Adequate audiological and educational diagnosis and assessment* of the child such that any decisions made for programming are based upon sound information which is to be shared with all those involved in the child's education.

2. *Comprehensive information from tests.* The audiologist who fails to report to teachers because "They can't understand the information" is revealing a personal weakness rather than that of the teacher. Teachers want to do the best for the children under their care. Time should be set aside for examination of all findings of relevance to the teacher, and educational implications discussed with the teacher. Results are best reported to teachers in a profile manner, using the context of age performances and grade equivalencies.

3. *In-service training* should be planned for about 2 days at the onset of the school year and provided for all teachers who will be working with hearing-impaired children.* This training should include appropriate college credit as incentive and should ensure a basic understanding of hearing loss, hearing aids, room arrangement, acoustics, support services available, legal responsibilities, reading materials, etc.
4. *Ongoing support* is required from the educational audiologist to monitor progress, and to ensure that teachers are making maximum use of services available. Given the appropriate support, things do happen, and all those concerned will be less negative towards the experience. Ongoing support is also needed to encourage appropriate hearing aid and FM usage and to encourage appropriate classroom situations.
5. There is a need for introduction of a *trouble-shooting program* for audiological equipment which is easily maintained by the teacher and/or the child and overseen by the educational audiologist. Support in initiating this program as well as offering ideas for making it routine, as well as offering a good repair and return service, helps the audiological service appear operational.
6. Above all, teachers need *excellent supervision and support* from the administration. They need *advice* on who can best provide for the child's needs. The educational audiologist should be in a position to access teachers of the deaf for academic tutoring and speechreading, to access speech-language pathologists for remediation of deviances and psychologists, and others for their particular competencies. Teachers need *help* in modifying their style of teaching to accomodate the hard-of-hearing child. This takes time and demands sensitive interactions between the classroom teacher and the supervisor. Authoritative, teacher-centered, whole-class teaching methods rarely work when individuals have unusual needs.
7. *Periodic workshops/conferences* for teachers and support staff are an excellent idea. In Utah, an Educational Audiology Workshop is held each year to which teachers, audiologists, speech pathologists, and administrators are invited to hear a speaker on current issues of importance to the management of the hard-of-hearing child in the classroom.

By establishing professional contact with teachers and support staff, and by offering their expertise in audiology along with their skills in coordination and leadership, educational audiologists make themselves accessible.

Facilitating Teacher Growth

The 10 techniques described by Glickman (1981) provide good suggestions for educational audiologists to use in their planned improvement in communication with teachers. These are worthy of examination at length. By

---

*L. Van Dyke, personal communication, July 28, 1984.

implementing these strategies, educational audiologists can make effective contact, develop an understanding and follow through on needs and problems.

The first technique for facilitating growth is *good listening.* The primary task is to let the teacher talk. Too often, teachers perceive that their ideas and feelings are never listened to and that they have limited value. Letting teachers share feelings and attitudes produces tremendous affirmation to the teacher. This is always followed by *clarifying* what is being said. Reiterating the ideas expressed by teachers will let them know that what is being said is understood correctly. This technique greatly enhances the communication interchange.

A third technique is *encouragement.* Teachers often feel that a person coming into their room is judgmental. The teacher has feeling of being evaluated and criticized. When this feeling of evaluation is present, the classroom teacher is defensive and is often unable to communicate openly and honestly. The educational audiologist must therefore be prepared to encourage teachers to talk about their concerns, fears, and frustrations. It is also effective for the educational audiologist to honestly encourage the teacher to continue doing something that is important. Each person needs to know he is doing something of worth, and it is a valuable lesson in management to always find something supportive to say about others.

Another skill is the ability to *express* educational suggestions as an outgrowth of the teacher's expressed concerns. We all learn the most when we see a need to learn and when we want to learn. For example, it is quite probable that teachers will feel uncomfortable with hearing aids and other types of amplification. The first task is to help the teacher talk about the problem. The conversation may go something like this; "How is Peter's hearing aid working?" The usual response is: "Fine." All too frequently, the initial statement is accepted without the listener really determining what is meant. A way to check on how the teacher really feels is to ask specific closed questions: "Did the batteries register all right this morning?" This specific question may reveal some problems or concerns that the teacher has about checking batteries. Through the teacher's questions, the educational audiologist will gain the knowledge necessary for providing a meaningful impact.

The time spent evaluating problems and needs, or *problem solving,* is essential to ongoing improvement. The primary task is to identify problems. This is an outgrowth of the conversations and interactions that the educational audiologist has had with the teacher. The problems will begin to emerge as the educational audiologist spends time with the teacher, using many of the procedures described above. Once a problem has been identified, the procedure is to first explore what has been done to solve it and to then make suggestions concerning what might be tried. The suggestions must be those which can be easily accommodated within the scope of the teacher's work, and which will not be perceived as more added to an already overburdened schedule.

In order to successfully accomplish the task described above, a sixth technique will frequently need to be used, that of *negotiation.* The teacher

and the educational audiologist need to discuss possible ways to solve problems and then need to negotiate a practical solution agreed to by both
professionals. It may be necessary to determine some joint tasks that can be
performed. It is important to remember, however, that the changes will likely
be small in the beginning, and it is important not to expect a complete change
overnight. Change is only possible when someone perceives a need for
change. The educational audiologist may see a glaring problem that must be
changed, but if the teacher cannot perceive the problem, the possibility for
change is very small at the outset.

The teacher may be helped to perceive a problem through the use of
demonstration. Again, the process must be one where the teacher agrees
that the demonstration might be useful. Once it is agreed that the educational
audiologist should demonstrate something, the activity is planned together
so that the teacher sees the whole process from planning through implementation. This aids in building collaboration and cooperation. People who
do things together, who talk together and share concerns, tend to grow in
positive ways.

A technique which is often selected by educational audiologists is that
of *direct guidance* to the teacher. This process usually involves providing the
teacher with a fairly lengthy list of suggestions to be followed when there are
hearing-impaired children in the classroom. Without the concurrent use of
many of the other techniques described above, this procedure is very ineffective. A teacher typically will not remember the 20-item list and may, in fact,
feel resentment at being given suggestions. At best, the teacher will remember
one or two of the ideas and file the rest in a folder for later reference. By
spending time with individual teachers, educational audiologists will learn
how to best approach them with information. A personalized, shortened list
for each specific child is a successful strategy.

Standardization can only be used when the teacher is seeking assistance. In this instance, the teacher believes that some changes need to be
made, but does not know what they are. The educational audiologist offers
to observe and collect baseline data on some of the areas of concern. The
teacher and the educational audiologist agree on the observation and, after
the data are collected, they examine them together and agree on what needs
to be changed and standards for improvement are then selected and agreed
upon. Data should be reanalyzed after intervention has occurred and each
teacher is then provided with further feedback on the success of the change
decided upon previously and to their possible future involvement with hearing
impaired students.

The last technique of *reinforcement* is used in conjunction with standardization, as described above. This process involves providing feedback on
the progress made toward objectives agreed upon. There may be 20 areas
of concern, but the introduction of each should be prioritized and each should
be reinforced at regular intervals. One of the teacher's greatest needs is to

have a sense that what they are doing is appropriately and well done. The educational audiologist can function as a provider of positive feedback to the teacher. This technique is very powerful in bringing about change.

The use of these 10 techniques will have a significant, positive impact on teachers and will also, as a consequence, improve services to the hearing impaired. The biggest single problem in using the techniques is the lack of time most educational audiologist have available. When the average educational audiologist has responsibility for a large school district, or for 2 or 3 large schools, time becomes very limited. Under the present conditions, the implementation of all procedures described in this book is therefore not possible. It is necessary for the educational audiologist to make significant changes in the system if appropriate services are to be provided. Changing the any system takes time, however.

Some individuals working within a school system suggest that the average time necessary to make meaningful change is from 3 to 5 years. Any change is gradual and, in many instances, it takes longer than 5 years before full implementation of a new program can be realized. On the other hand, it is also clear that systems tend to maintain the status quo as long as there is no perceived reason to change. If teachers are to change, they must see new alternatives to the practices they now use. They must feel the school leadership is enthusiastic and knowledgeable about the new practices and is supportive of them. Planned change would involve school leaders providing consultants or speakers in school audiology, in-service training for teachers, and materials, all as a means of showing their support. Educational audiologists are advised to develop annual goals for change and to analyze their progress several times during the year. If educational audiologists realize there are stages of change in the improvement process, they can begin to work towards implementation with all involved.

IMPLEMENTING THE DELIVERY OF SERVICES MODEL

One of the hardest decisions faced by educational audiologists interested in implementing change is that of where to begin. What become the priority areas amenable to change? Which decisions will guarantee success? These are vital questions which need to be answered if the service delivery is to be enhanced.

The first step in change initiation is deciding what parts of the Model Delivery of Services (Fig. 8-2) are currently being implemented and which parts should make up a full-time responsibility for the educational audiologist. An examination of the typical workload will require some soul-searching questions. Will change require a modification of the time allocations of personnel doing the job? Is time well organized? Is time well spent? Is travel time coordinated? Any number of situations may leave room for change and allow

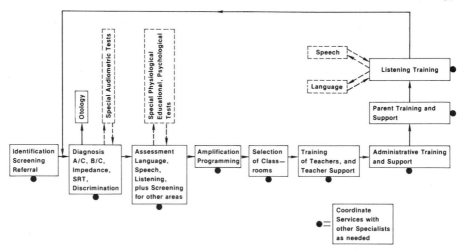

Fig. 8-2. Model of delivery of educational audiology services. The solid lines indicate that the educational audiologist will be directly involved with these activities. The dotted lines suggest that the educational audiologist may be involved either directly or indirectly with these services.

time for additional services. The important thing is to be critical of the role responsibilities. A possible approach is to begin by completing a time analysis over several months to identify areas of current focus.

It is worthwhile to select an area for change which will provide a high degree of success. Although all change takes time (years in many cases), there are small changes which can be made on a regular basis.

Identification, Screening, and Referral

Most educational audiologists undertake screening of students as part of their audiological service in schools. For many, this is a very time-consuming routine task, taking many weeks to complete. It is basically a technical task, and, if carried out by a technician, leaves the master's level audiologist free to pursue the more complex elements of the job and to introduce new areas of responsibility. There are volunteer groups of parents and nurses who may be trained, coordinated, and supervised by the educational audiologist to do the types of screening required, although close supervision and evaluation of technical staff is mandatory. The necessity for above-average technical and interpersonal skills on the part of the educational audiologist becomes obvious. An educational audiologist's direct involvement will ultimately depend on agency numbers and the extent of the screening process, but it can be a delegated job and will free time for other tasks.

Diagnosic Audiometry

Diagnostic audiometry will continue to be a primary area of responsibility for educational audiologists. The question becomes one of what tests should be provided and one of accountability: "Do we test and obtain results indicating deficiencies when there are no programs to help the child?" The debate regarding special tests is particularly relevant here. What do audiologists discover from those tests and what are the educational implications for such findings? To date, audiologists have been notoriously deficient in knowing what to do with their special test results. Traditionally, the results are filed and the problems left to an unknowledgeable teacher to solve. Above all, the audiologist must be responsible for coordinating test results and providing an interpretation of how they relate to classroom and learning styles.

Assessment

The importance of assessment, along with a detailed account of tests available, was covered in Chapter 3, in which the PEMICS Model of developmental assessment is discussed. The need for accurate, helpful information gathered during the assessment process must be emphasized. While educational audiologists are not seen as being responsible for all testing, it is recommended that they collate the information to ensure comprehensive reporting and dissemination of the findings. An ideal opportunity for coordination of services exists here. It is true that educational audiologists have had little, if any, training in this area in the past, nor, it appears, have they expressed much interest (Wilson-Vlotman. 1984). Seeking collaboration with resource room teachers, teachers of the deaf, psychologists, learning disability LD specialists, and speech-language pathologists, and pooling information will enhance service delivery to the child. What has been historically absent is the coordination of information by a case manager for hearing-impaired students. Educational audiologists should take this responsibility and set up profiles to enhance parent and professional understanding of the findings from the assessment process.

Amplification Programming

Surprisingly, only 10 percent of educational audiologists view themselves as primarily responsible for the day-to-day monitoring of hearing aids in schools (Wilson-Vlotman, 1984). If they are not monitoring, it is likely no one is. Regular classroom teachers are not well enough trained, nor have much time for amplification issues. Teachers of the deaf have not undertaken this role as a primary function. Educational audiologists must see this as a primary function if the maximization of residual hearing is the ultimate goal of audiology (which, of course, it is!). The question is who will monitor amplification, and what will that person do? Again, the job is one of establishing a sound program, training responsible persons, ensuring that the job is being done, and providing a speedy repair service when problems are identified. There always will be hearing aids and FM units to repair!

Training for optimal use of amplification equipment in a school setting is also the educational audiologist's responsibility and must be built into the schedule when a new child enters the program or new teachers become involved.

Classroom Selection

There are many structurally inappropriate classrooms in our schools today. (Chapter 7 deals with this issue). The room location may have a poor signal-to-noise ratio, the lighting and furnishings and room arrangement may be unsatisfactory. These are not uncontrollable factors if there is a committment to an optimal learning environment for the hearing-impaired child. For too long, however, such factors have been ignored. Hearing aids are of little value to the child if they are not functioning optimally. In electing a classroom placement for the child, the case manager must know conditions in the various classrooms and must take into account the amount of support the selected teacher will need in order to overcome the remaining adverse conditions. It is encouraging to learn that some audiology programs recognize a need in this area and are beginning to instruct students accordingly. Educational audiologists should also have input into new schools planned for their districts by suggesting possible acoustical treatment of classrooms, facilities for special testing, and basic equipment required. Creating satisfactory conditions for the maximum use of students' residual hearing is not a simple task—yet it is basic to a child's successful educational program.

Training of Teachers and Teacher Support

As noted in Chapter 2, educational audiologists across the nation have a seemingly distant relationship with teachers. Over half confer with teachers only 1–2 hours each week. Educational audiologists generally have extraordinarily large caseloads of children. They often feel comfortable in their relationship with teachers, even though they do not indicate respect for the teachers' skills in handling the hearing-impaired child (Wilson-Vlotman, 1984). Disparity exists here, for many educational audiologists indicate little commitment to education or a positive attitude about their school role (Wilson-Vlotman, 1984). As noted mutual respect between the educational audiologist and teachers must precede meaningful change. Educational audiologists must spend time with teachers both formally in in-service training and informally whenever possible. They must provide an office telephone number and office hours to facilitate quick and easy communication. Building this as a role of an educational audiologist indicates an positive commitment to change.

Administrative Training and Support

Time is well spent finding out about, and communicating with key decision-makers. Means to accomplish this are discussed in a later section in this chapter.

Parent Training and Support

Parents are an untapped source and support system. Means to involve them and foster advocacy are discussed below.

Listening Training and Other Direct Services

Of the direct service activities of the educational audiologists sampled in the national study, listening (auditory) training is the most popular—38 percent of all educational audiologists questioned focused on that aspect of aural rehabilitation. (Wilson-Vlotman, 1984). Other aural (re)habilitative activities are far less likely to be part of a program of aural (re)habilitation. Someone must be seen as responsible for listening training. (See Chapter 6 for a discussion of state-of-the-art listening training.) If the educational audiologist is to be involved in any direct service provisions, listening training seems the most appropriate. The decisions to be made are related to when and to whom will it be delivered and what form will it take. The question of other aural (re)habilitative services (speech, reading, language, and academics) is a decision involving questions of time, skill, need, and other support services available. To adequately meet the total management needs of the hearing-impaired child, direct services seem the most dispensible area for an educational audiologist. It was the least popular responsibility of all educational audiologists questioned, the responsibility for which they felt least qualified. If an educational audiologist, as a child's case manager, undertakes to coordinate direct services appropriate to a child's needs and to ensure that those needs are being met, that audiologist is free to begin change in the audiological service. Excessive direct service responsibility is extremely time-consuming and its value to the overall success or failure of a program should be analyzed carefully.

The above suggestions focus upon the educational audiologist as a case manager for hearing-handicapped children in regular school placement. The focus of the job is on coordination and public relations as well as on audiological skill. Such a role demands a greater maturity in leadership and public school management than is currently the case. The challenge for exellence and planned change is before the audiologist in the school.

SUPPORTING AND TRAINING PARENTS

It is unfortunate that most parents of a hard-of-hearing child have been subject to constant humiliation by professionals (Schulz, 1985). They not only lack information relative to the consequences of hearing loss of varying degree, but may also develop many negative attitudes about their child, attitudes borne of isolation, confusion, and fear. Parents who harbor fears that their child is "different" are often reluctant to seek professional advice. In recognizing their child is not developing age-appropriate communication skills, they may regard their child as being noncompliant or as having cognitive deficits—unless they have sought out adequate professional consultation. Many parents of young hearing-impaired children have reported that they stopped talking because the child did not respond, or because when the child does talk, speech is unintelligible. Parents of young children who have been identified as hearing impaired are counseled to talk to their children even if the children do not respond (Clark & Watkins, 1985).

To develop coping strategies, many parents need some form of counseling. Parents must be helped to deal with feelings associated with the handicap; they must be helped to understand the processes involved in hearing, listening, and speech, and how they each relate to the ability to learn. Parent-infant programs have a definite place in aiding and supporting parents and should meet their need to understand normal development as well as to understand how to enjoy their child. In general, parental needs are emotionally based for a long time and are determined by the stages of crisis through which the individual is passing at a certain time. Educational audiologists are in a position as case managers to ensure that parents have support groups and contact with other needed support services available.

Successfully mainstreaming any hearing-impaired child necessitates that all personnel work towards this goal. Parents should be encouraged to become involved in the educational process, as the degree of success of the child depends to a great extent upon parental support of the program. Yet, how often are parents considered to be a hindrance to educational programming for their child? Traditionally, parents have been excluded from school involvement, particularly as their children get older. No school program can be fully effective without carryover into the home. Knowledgeable and supportive parents provide a positive addition to any educational planning. The development of the Individualized Educational Plan (IEP), in which decisions involve the parents, along with the professional support of team members, are made based on the child's educational needs and has been a very positive step in the education of handicapped children.

As both diagnosticians and environmental managers, educational audiologists are in a unique position. They have the knowledge relating to hearing necessary to undertake the responsibility to educate parents and professionals about the impact of hearing loss on the total child. They must accept the challenge of being informed of appropriate support services available to parents and must recognize the fact that they have a principal role to play in the management of the hearing-impaired child. This role must be well defined. The educational audiologist, as the diagnostician, is often the first person to identify a hearing loss and first to inform the parents. In a recent study, educational audiologists in the United States indicated that their principal contacts with parents were when conducting hearing assessments and/ or at IEP meetings (Wilson-Vlotman, 1984). It is encouraging to know that they are making contact with parents, but the extent of the contact and the attitude towards it is not known, although it is not seen to be continually supportive, considering the brief nature of the contact. How this initial contact is handled will probably be an important factor determining the progress the entire family makes in accepting and managing the handicap. To inform parents of the loss and to then assume that another person will deal with the management of that loss is a poor but prevailing practice of (educational) audiologists generally, and is, at the very least, unprofessional. In the managerial role, the educational audiologist is responsible for discussing test results with parents, making referrals where necessary, making recommendations for placement, and working closely with parents, teachers, and administrators in following through. By the time recommendations are to be made, the educational audiologist ideally should have established a trusting relationship with the parents (Stream & Stream, 1978).

The most fundamental lesson to be learned by any professional is that parents are people too, and that they are primarily responsible for their child's welfare. While professionals and parents have worked together, traditionally there has been conflict (Schulz, 1985). Historically, parents have lacked trust in professionals, who tend to view themselves as providing services which are not to be questioned. Educational audiologists must refrain from falling into this trap if they are to earn the support of parents in initiating change in service options to hearing-handicapped, mainstreamed children.

All professionals must ask themselves how they view parents. Are they seen as being either overprotective or uncaring? Are they seen as a hindrance to getting a job done? What is their place in the school setting? Why is it parents don't seem to care about the work professionals (teachers and specialists) do for their children? It has been the writer's experience that there are many valid reasons why parents react the way they do towards their children's school program. These reasons need to be understood before effective interaction may proceed.

> Two factors [seem] crucial to effective parent-professional interaction: communication and respect. While these elements are essential to any good relationship, they seem to be missing in many of our parent-teacher (professional) confrontations. (Schulz, 1985, p. 5)

Stream & Stream (1978, ch. 9 1981) outline 4 goals for an audiologist in working with parents:

1. Present information on the child's hearing as it relates to factors that can affect the child's learning potential.

2. Develop realistic supportive educational plans for school or for special programs within the home.
3. Support parents in dealing with their feelings relative to their problems associated with the handicap.
4. Allow parents to enhance their general understanding and acceptance of the hearing impairment.

To which should be added:

5. Train parents to fully understand the purpose and use of acoustical equipment recommended for their child.
6. Encourage parents to be consistent, skilled observers of their child's progress and development, and provide information which will help them to understand the child in the environment as a whole.
7. Set up a parental network of concerned and knowledgeable parents who can assist new parents of hearing-impaired children.
8. Set up an open house, display annual statistics, and organize activities.
9. Ask parents for their help and guide them regarding the many ways they can help make the audiological program visible and indispensible. If parents receive the services they need, they will provide an excellent support system. Visibility is achieved by letters of support to key decision-makers, membership on committees, and involvement in advocacy programs.

The educational audiologist who functions as a manager of children's hearing has a challenging task. Above all else, parents must be helped to become advocates for their children throughout their school days. Parents need the support of a professional who can provide guidance and direction to sources of support and education while understanding the total dimension of the hearing handicap.

TRAINING AND INVOLVING ADMINISTRATORS

The administration is the key factor to effective implementation of any school program. The study by Wilson-Vlotman (1984) revealed that educational audiologists are concerned about the fact that administrators misunderstand their job and view them as having very narrow role responsibilities related to diagnosis and assessment. Audiologists feel they lack support, which undercuts their ability to function effectively in their job. Educational audiologists feel unappreciated by their administrators. Appreciation comes from awareness, and if administrators are unfamiliar with the audiological service and its value, this alone may have led to a great deal of the job dissatisfaction reported in the study of educational audiology in the United States (Wilson-Vlotman, 1984).

Sarnecky (1981b) noted 3 barriers to effective program implementation by audiologists in schools:

1. Audiologists are unfamiliar with the administration of the public school.
2. School personnel are unfamiliar with role and responsibilities of the school audiologist.
3. School personnel do not understand the characteristics and needs of hearing-impaired children.

One barrier Sarnecky (1981b) did not discuss, but which became apparent through the Wilson-Vlotman (1984) study, was:

4. Educational audiologists are inadequately trained in organizational theory, which deters them from effectively managing the residual hearing of the hard-of-hearing child.

To be fully functioning, any system needs all components of that system operating well. Educational audiologists who have excellent clinical skills and yet who have no idea of how to transfer that information to the classroom, and who ignore the needs of the administration for efficacy, visibility and essentiality, may find themselves at the very least dissatisfied and ineffective, and may be even out of a job as money is directed to more visible areas.

How can the administration become more aware of the educational audiologists and the services they provide in their schools? A specialty area is only as strong as its advocates, and educational audiologists should view public relations as a continuing responsibility of the job. They must learn to become visible. The administration is not always at fault. Change is always need-related and educational audiologists must be able to explain the value of an audiological service based in a school district. Diagnosis and assessment of hearing loss alone do not warrant the cost involved in such a service.

The personnel in administration with whom the educational audiologist must become familiar and from whom support must be solicited include: the superintendent and principal, who are responsible for budget, program efficacy, and public relations in a school district; the key decision-makers in the schools, whose identity may be quite surprising and who may not always be the principal; and, program coordinators who are the supervisors and program evaluators. It should not be assumed that any one of these individuals knows anything of the specialty area the audiologist supervises; these individuals may not be informed advocates.

How to Train Administrators and Key Personnel

The administration must come to believe in the educational audiology service as an integral part of its school program; this is achieved through continued awareness. There are many ways to ensure that this exposure occurs:

1. Keep statistics of children seen, types of problems encountered, etc. This allows the use of these data in support of the case for increased resources and in summary reports. Data do talk!

2. Write a role description of the job and have it available for discussion. Complete a monthly time analysis of the job. A good guide here is the model of educational audiology referred to in the beginning of this book. It is often somewhat startling to see how much time is being spent in the numerous facets of one's job. Keep in mind that the ideal caseload is 5000–8000 students. Not many work in such luxury, so it is important that a decision be made regarding what parts of the Model of Delivery of Audiological Service will be the focus while work goes ahead to institute change in numbers, services, and staff.†

3. Have parents write letters of support to key persons (superintendent, principal, and immediate supervisor) for audiological services, indicating the importance to them of such services.

4. Volunteer to speak to parent groups. Have organizers write letters of thanks to the superintendent.

5. Speak to community groups. Have letters of thanks written to key personnel.

6. Present papers at local and national meetings and have announcements of meetings mailed to supervisors

7. Agree to supervise trainees. Have letters of support written from the training institutions.

8. Make contact with support persons in the community who may help provide a better service to the school through equipment donations.

9. Become familiar with all support persons available in the school district. Invite them to speak at meetings, observe their programs, and periodically elicit their expertise.

10. Write annual reports of program activities and distribute these to key personnel. This not only provides information to the administration but enables an evaluation of the program services and a subsequent re-working of program goals.

11. Organize workshops for staff; invite key personnel and support persons. Effective change assumes all involved have a sound knowledge base. Be prepared to give time to organization and presentation at these workshops. This is time-consuming, but worth it.

12. If working between schools, *always* announce arrivals and departures from schools to the secretary and principal, if appropriate. Visibility is gained when others are aware of timetables, of when to expect the audiologist and where the audiologist will be.

13. Make informal contact with teachers. This will help in decisions regard-

---

† L. Van Dyke, personal communication, July 28, 1984.

ing placement of students as the audiologist is able to make knowledgeable judgments of staff available in a school. The staffroom is an excellent place for incidental contacts, where the audiologist can be available to talk with teachers and others about their problems and plans. It will take time to feel comfortable, as the audiologist is only there occasionally, but perseverance will bring rewards.

14. Be positive, find good in people, gain their trust.
15. Be aware of the inherent hierarchy of responsibilities found in schools. Include immediate supervisors in plans and try to avoid sidestepping them when trying to get things done. Sidestepping creates barriers.
16. Learn about various leadership styles and about how to influence people. Work out the leadership styles of your school administrators and learn to work with them.
17. Know the legislation concerning the hearing impaired so that actions can be defended from a legal stand point. Interpret legislation for others and bring about change.
18. Use the news media to have stories done on the children. School boards love publicity!

Above all, ensure that the program is visible and provides an indispensible service. Bureaucratic systems are complex and schools are no exception. To someone without an awareness of how organizational hierarchies function, understanding how to go about change in schools will be difficult. The educational audiologist would be well advised to seek some training in the area. It takes time to develop skills, to become known and appreciated by one's peers, and to create an irreplacable service—but it can be done.

SUMMARY

Educational audiology has become an essential service in schools. Foregoing chapters in this book laid the foundations for recommended audiological provisions to hard-of-hearing children in the mainstreamed setting, while this chapter considered the role of the educational audiologist in providing a total management service. It is not satisfactory for a school-based audiologist to provide only diagnostics and assessment, for this can be completed in any clinic-based setting. The uniqueness of educational audiologists is their skill in using test information from a variety of sources available to schools to the best advantage of the hearing-impaired student. The educational audiologist should have an understanding of the educational, social, and emotional needs of the child and should involve parents, teachers, and administrators in meeting these needs. By learning how to best work with these 3 groups, the educational audiologist will have the advocates needed to initiate change in the delivery of audiological services in schools.

Educational audiologists have much to learn and achieve in the school setting. There are increasing numbers of educational audiologists as more and more universities and school districts seek to fill audiological positions with people who have had more training and experience than are available in the narrowly focused clinical programs. These audiologists have the responsibility to begin to formalize and consolidate their position professionally. As noted previously, many educational audiologists are unhappy with their perceived second-rate status and fail to take the responsibility for their careers. Ways of dealing with this have been alluded to in this chapter and others; they involve fundamental organizational leadership issues, including:

1. Ensuring job expertise;
2. Engaging in professional education and training—implying leadership and supervisory skills as well as knowledge of how a school functions (Berg, 1982);
3. Seeking opportunities for professional interchange through networking as more people enter the field;
4. Formalizing rules, procedures, and policies which provide functional and operational guidelines for the profession.

Educational audiology is no longer in its infancy. A model of delivery of services has been proposed throughout the book, based upon an extensive national study of full-time educational audiologists (Wilson-Vlotman, 1984), as well as a comprehensive fault-tree analysis of competencies within the field. Educational audiologists are challenged to evaluate their current service programs in light of these recommendations.

REFERENCES

American Speech-Language-Hearing Association. Audiology services in the schools position statement. *ASHA,* 1983, *25*(5), 53–60.

Berg F S. *Special project doctoral program hearing impaired educational audiology resource,* Final report, Grant Number G007900861 Logan, Utah: Utah State University, 1982.

Bess F H & McConnell F E. *Audiology, education, and the hearing impaired child.* Chapter 8, Missouri: C. V. Mosby, 1981.

Blair J C & Berg F S. Problems and needs of hard-of-hearing students and a model of delivery of services to schools. *ASHA,* 1982, 24(8), 541–546.

Campbell R F, Cunningham L L, Nystrand R D, & Usdan M D. *The organization and control of American schools* (4th ed.). Columbus, Ohio: Charles E. Merrill, 1980.

Clark T C & Watkins S. *Programming for hearing impaired infants through amplification and home intervention.* Logan, Utah: Ski*Hi Institute 1985.

Doll R C. *Supervision for staff development: Ideas and application.* Boston: Allyn and Bacon, Inc., 1983.

Garstecki D C. Survey of school audiologists. *ASHA,* 1978, *20*(4), 291–296.

Garwood V P. Audiological management of the hearing impaired child in the public schools. In F N Martin (Ed.), *Pediatric audiology* Englewood Cliffs, N. J.: Prentice-Hall, 1978.

Glickman C D. *Developmental Supervision,* Association for Supervision and Curriculum Development. Alexandria, Va., 1981.

Hoversten G H. A public school audiology program: Amplification, maintenance, auditory management and inservice education. In F H Bess, B A Freeman, & J S Sinclair (Eds.), *Amplification in education.* Washington, D.C.: Alexander Graham Bell Association for the Deaf, 1980, pp. 224–267.

Lewin K. Group decision and social change. In T Newcomb & E Hartely (Eds.), *Readings in social psychology.* New York: Holt Rinehart & Winston, 1947.

Lieberman, A & Miller L. *Teachers, their world and their work. Implications for school improvement.* Alexandria, Va.: Association for Supervision and Curriculum Development, 1984 Ch 5.

Ross M. The audiologist in the schools. *ASHA,* 1979, *21*(9), 858–860.

Ross M & Calvert D R. Guidelines for audiology programs in educational settings for hearing impaired children. *Volta Review,* 1977, *79,* 153–161.

Sarnecky, E A. *Audiologists in school settings: Preparation and functions.* Unpublished doctoral dissertation, Washington, DC, Gallaudet College, 1982.

Sarnecky, E A. Eliminating barriers to successful implementation of audiology programs in schools. *Hearing Aid Journal,* July 1981, pp. 4; 36–38.

Schulz J B. The Parent-Professional conflict. In Turnbull & Turnbull. *Parents speak out.* San Diego: College Hill Press, 1985.

Szilagyi A D & Wallace M J. *Organizational behavior and performance* (2nd ed.). Santa Monica: Goodyear Publishing Company, 1980.

Stream R W & Stream K S. Counseling the parents of the hearing-impaired child. In F Martin (Ed.), *Pediatric Audiology.* New Jersey: Prentice Hall, Inc., 1978.

U.S. House of Representatives, Conference Report. *Education of handicapped children,* Report no. 94–664. Washington, D.C., November 14, 1975.

Wilson-Vlotman A L. *Educational audiology: Practices, attitudes and organizational structures.* Unpublished doctoral dissertation, Utah State University, 1984.

Yater V Y. Educational audiology. In J Katz (Ed.), *Handbook of clinical audiology* (2nd ed.). Baltimore: Williams & Wilkins, 1978.

Index